Introduction to ophthalmoscopy

A SCOPE® PUBLICATION

David Paton, MD, FACS
Professor and Chairman
Department of Ophthalmology
Baylor College of Medicine

Barry N. Hyman, MD
Assistant Professor
Department of Ophthalmology
Baylor College of Medicine
and
The Zimmerman Medical Clinic

Johnny Justice, Jr.
Assistant Professor
Department of Ophthalmology
Baylor College of Medicine

Published by The Upjohn Company, Kalamazoo, Michigan

Upjohn

4

Editor Emeritus/Baird A. Thomas

8801-12R

TABLE OF CONTENTS

6

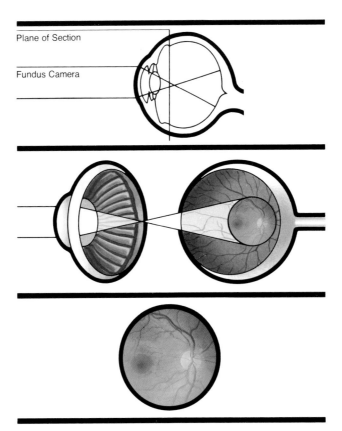

Plane of Section

Fundus Camera

Figure 1. Fundus photographs reveal only a small portion of the entire retina (see page 13). Most of the color illustrations in this book demonstrate abnormalities of the posterior fundus, generally in the vicinity of the optic nerve head and posterior pole. Some of the illustrations show lesions at the equator of the eye and a few that are more peripheral. It is important to realize that fundus pathology is often diffuse, that multiple lesions may co-exist, and that many of the most significant abnormalities of the retina lie further peripheral than the range of the direct ophthalmoscope and the fundus camera.

Preface

It is the purpose of this monograph to teach the beginner some of the fundamentals of ophthalmoscopy. That sentence was used by Dan M. Gordon, M.D. introducing a monograph of the same nature published by The Upjohn Company. The intention of the present authorship remains the same. The monograph now presented is totally rewritten and all but six of the illustrations are new. We have covered much of the same material and in a similar sequence as that selected by the late Dr. Gordon. We are presenting a unique series of fundus illustrations that have been carefully selected for their technical excellence and teaching value. These photographs were selected from patient case files collected at the Department of Ophthalmology of Baylor College of Medicine, the Wilmer Institute of The Johns Hopkins Hospital, the National Institute of Neurological Diseases and Blindness (predecessor of the National Eye Institute), the Bascom Palmer Eye Institute of the University of Miami, and the Wills Eye Institute in Philadelphia.

This monograph is only a first step in teaching the diagnosis of fundus abnormalities. Many of the illustrated disorders of the retina, choroid, and optic nerve discussed in this text have been selected primarily *to demonstrate representative examples of the spectrum of ocular fundus abnormalities.* Thus, we have chosen some esoteric lesions as well as many others that are rather common.

We are grateful to the publishers for permitting us to provide a completely new monograph and for their preoccupation in assuring high quality color reproductions. The aggregate number of copies of the preceding monograph that were printed and distributed in its five years of existence was exceedingly great. Perhaps this new issue will have similar distribution; if so, we hope that it will fulfill its teaching purposes. We anticipate the opportunity of improving future editions by receiving criticism and suggestions. There is always some risk of oversimplification in a short text, but it will serve effectively if it provides motivation for future learning.

David Paton, MD, FACS
Barry N. Hyman, MD
Johnny Justice, Jr.

8

Figure 2. The *direct ophthalmoscope* can be used with the patient in the sitting or supine position. Depending upon the refractive error of the examiner, glasses may be worn or removed. For examination of the optic nerve head, the patient's gaze should be fixed straight ahead and the examiner's gaze directed along an axis slightly nasal to the visual axis of the patient's eye.

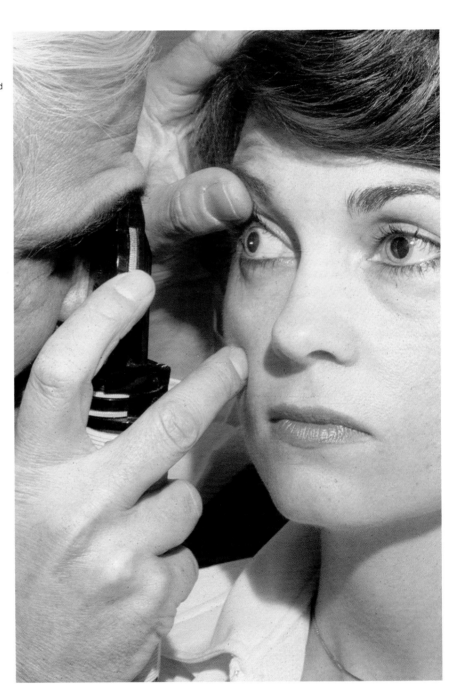

The Ophthalmoscopes

The ophthalmoscope (Figure 2) is one of the most important instruments in the diagnosis of disease. The information obtained from its use is dependent upon the quality of the instrument and the expertise of the user. The best hand instruments are those that connect to "house current" via a transformer yielding a 12-volt power supply. This gives a strong light source, optimal for direct ophthalmoscopy. Most battery-powered ophthalmoscopes operate on two volts; the light, however, is sufficient for the average purpose and the instrument is conveniently portable. It is well to remember always to employ fresh (or freshly charged) batteries when using the battery-powered ophthalmoscopes so as to obtain maximal light.

The bespectacled examiner may wish to use the ophthalmoscope while wearing his own eyeglasses. For this purpose, there is a rubber guard on the instrument head to prevent any lens scratches. The *direct ophthalmoscope's* head contains a rotary disc with a series of plus and minus lenses ranging up to 15 or 20 diopters of power. Myopia (nearsightedness) is neutralized ophthalmoscopically by the minus lenses (red numbers) and hyperopia (farsightedness) by the plus lenses (black numbers) of the ophthalmoscope. Instruments that connect to a transformer contain accessory discs of viewing lenses to provide as much as 40 diopters of lens power. If one is examining the fundus of a patient who wears a very high-minus lens, it may be helpful to do so through the patient's glasses, thus permitting the use of a low-power lens in the ophthalmoscope. This procedure is not advisable in viewing "high-plus fundi" of aphakic individuals. (Aphakia means without a lens – as when the lens has been removed surgically.) Viewing the fundus through a patient's high-plus spectacle lens creates too much distortion.

Most hand ophthalmoscopes have devices to modify the projected light beam. These include two round apertures, a slit, a grid, and a green filter. The small and large *apertures* of the ophthalmoscope are intended for small and large pupils, respectively. The vertical *slit* is for gauging convexity or concavity of a retinal lesion. When viewed with the slit beam, one of three impressions will be gained: (1) a flat lesion such as a hemorrhage, plaque, or scar will not distort the slit; (2) an elevated lesion such as a tumor or fibrous mass will, when the slit is placed over both it and the apparently normal retina, cause step-like distortion of the slit with the convexity toward the observer; and (3) a depressed area such as the excavation in the optic nerve, or a true hole in the macula (Figure 131) will, when the slit is placed over both the area surveyed and adjacent normal retina, cause the slit to be bowed away from the observer. (With the monocular direct ophthalmoscope, estimation of the convexity or concavity of a lesion is difficult.)

The *grid* can be used to measure vessel size by projecting the grid over the vessels and counting the number of spaces filled by a single vessel's caliber. The green *filter* provides a red-free light beam to help determine whether a black retinal "spot" is due to melanin or old hemorrhage. Unfortunately, the power (two volts) supplied by the battery-powered ophthalmoscope is often insufficient to accomplish this purpose. However, if the batteries are fresh, distinct benefit from the filter is obtained. With a red-free light of stronger voltage (ie, six to twelve volts), old hemoglobin appears coal black and melanin less black. Small aneurysms and hemorrhages, easily missed with ordinary two-volt illumination, stand out sharply (black in color) when the red-free light is employed. Obviously, the blood vessels will also stand out as black stripes with the red-free light. The use of red-free light helps to distinguish the normal nerve fibers of the retina coursing to the optic nerve (compare Figures 3 and 4). With optic atrophy, the nerve fibers are damaged and the super-

Figure 3. A normal right eye fundus. Notice the coloring of the optic nerve head and the central physiologic cupping constituting approximately one third of its area. Notice, too, the darker macular area in the horizontal meridian to the left of the optic nerve. The macula lies approximately 3 mm (2 disc diameters) temporal to the nerve head.

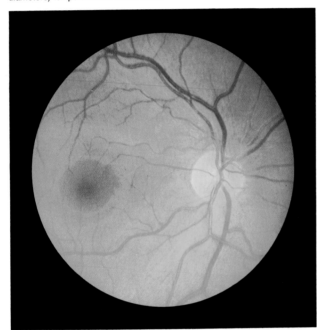

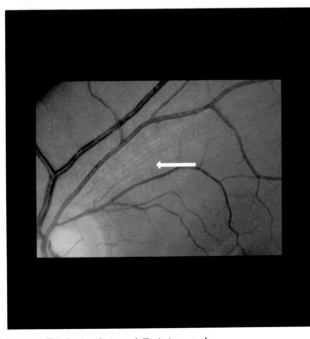

Figure 4. This fundus photograph illustrates use of the red-free light. Note the blackness of the vessels and the appearance of fine striations (arrow) at the level of the nerve fiber layer near the optic nerve head.

ficial retina may appear to have a marbled pattern. Whenever possible, the beginner should view the same fundus first through a battery-powered ophthalmoscope and then through a 12-volt instrument to demonstrate the advantages of the latter. Also be sure to try the green filter.

Dilatation of the pupil is necessary for a thorough examination of the fundus, although the pupils of most patients are large enough, and the lenses clear enough, to permit a satisfactory examination of the optic nerve heads and the surrounding retinal areas. Mydriasis is not to be confused with cycloplegia. Mydriasis simply means dilatation of the pupil; cycloplegia means not only pupillary dilatation but also drug-induced paralysis of the ciliary body. With cycloplegia, accommodation is paralyzed and the pupil will stay widely dilated when a strong examination light is employed – which is not the case if only mydriasis without cycloplegia has been induced with a sympathomimetic drug such as phenylephrine hydrochloride 10%. Cycloplegic agents are long-, intermediate-, and short-acting, and, for obvious reasons, it is advisable to use only short-acting cycloplegic agents such as tropicamide 0.5% or the 1% solution rather than long-acting cycloplegic agents such as atropine or homatropine. *It is common practice to obtain rapid mydriasis with cycloplegia, using a combination of phenylephrine hydrochloride 10% and tropicamide 0.5% by instilling each preparation several times in a 10-minute period.* Satisfactory dilatation of the pupil for examination with a strong light is usually obtained within 15 to 20 minutes. The effect of these eye drops is usually dissipated within two to four hours.

As stated, a thorough fundus examination cannot be performed without wide pupillary dilatation. The reasons for this will become more apparent later in the discussion. However, it is important to emphasize that many fundus examinations must be performed initially without the use of drops. Inequality of pupil size (dilatation or constriction of one or both pupils) and the speed of the pupils' response to light and to accommodation can all provide important diagnostic clues that should be evaluated before the use of eye drops. *Patients with recent head trauma or undiagnosed acute neurological disorders should not have dilated fundus examination under routine circumstances.*

There is another important reason why all pupils should not be dilated: the possibility of precipitating acute angle closure glaucoma. This form of glaucoma accounts for only 10% of glaucoma cases. It is confined almost exclusively to hyperopes (patients wearing plus or magnifying lenses), to patients of middle age or older, and to those whose eyes have a shallow anterior chamber. The examiner must estimate the depth of the chamber by handlight examination of all adult hyperopic patients considered for dilated fundus examination. When a handlight is directed obliquely at the eye, one soon learns to appraise the distance of the peripheral iris from the cornea near the limbus. If the iris appears close to the cornea, it should be considered to have a shallow chamber angle and, therefore, is an eye that may be dangerous to dilate. If the examiner can see that it is not shallow, the pupil can be dilated with confidence. If a slit lamp is unavailable, and should the examiner feel forced to dilate a potentially occludable angle, it is suggested that the patient receive a tablet of carbonic anhydrase inhibitor when dilatation is initiated and at least two successive instillations of pilocarpine 2% after the examination. The patient should be informed, in advance of the examination, about the possibility of inducing glaucoma. Further, the patient should be told that if pain or diminished vision ensues, an immediate succeeding ophthalmological examination will be mandatory.

Some physicians always employ pilocarpine subsequent to a dilated fundus examination. It is true that

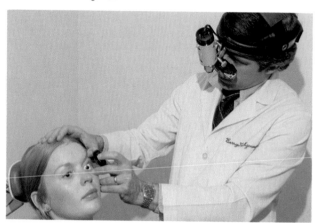

this probably speeds recovery of a more normal-sized pupil, thus providing more prompt return of normal visual function. Nevertheless, a low but significant incidence of retinal detachments has been reported following mydriasis terminated by drug-induced miosis. Therefore, many ophthalmologists do not employ pilocarpine routinely when the fundus examination has been completed.

The direct ophthalmoscope commonly employed by every physician is an indispensable instrument. The *binocular indirect ophthalmoscope*, however, affords a *stereoscopic* view of the entire fundus. It is worn on the observer's head and provides an illumined binocular viewing system (Figure 5). The image is produced by manipulation of an aspheric lens (called the loupe), held perpendicular to the illuminating light and at almost arm's length from the observer. Mastery of this technique requires not only special instruction but many hours of practice. To optimize indirect ophthalmoscopy, the patient's pupil *must* be widely dilated.

In general, the magnification of the direct ophthalmoscope is approximately 14 times the normal object size, whereas the indirect ophthalmoscope gives only 2 to 4x magnification, depending upon the power of the loupe. The direct ophthalmoscope gives a small field

Figure 6. This fundus painting demonstrates several important points. The entire retina is illustrated as though it were at a single plane. Actually, the circumference of the equator of the eye is considerably greater than that of the anterior margin of the peripheral retina; that margin (the ora) is shown in this rendition as the periphery of a large circle. Notice what a small portion of the fundus is occupied by the optic nerve and the posterior pole (macula). The painting depicts multiple abnormalities: a retinal detachment, subretinal tumor, chorioretinal scarring, and horseshoe-shaped retinal tear. The small circle illustrates the stereoscopic fundus view with the indirect ophthalmoscope as compared to the more magnified but much smaller area of fundus seen with the direct ophthalmoscope (shown within the small box to the right of the painting). Notice, too, that the image with the indirect ophthalmoscope is reversed and inverted. The extent of fundus photographed by the fundus camera constitutes a wider field of vision than provided with the direct ophthalmoscope, but considerably less than the field of vision with indirect ophthalmoscopy.

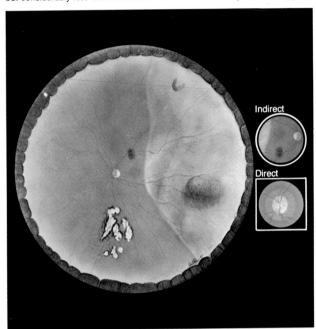

Indirect

Direct

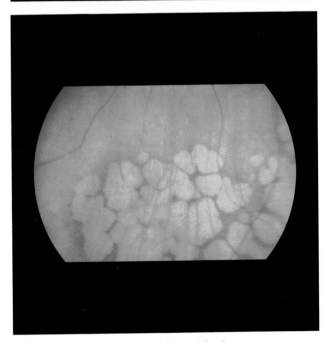

Figure 7. *Cobblestone degeneration* of the peripheral fundus is a benign abnormality of the aging eye. This condition is often difficult to see with the direct ophthalmoscope.

of approximately 10°, as compared to a 45° field with the indirect ophthalmoscope (Figure 6). By indenting the sclera with a scleral depressor, the examiner may visualize the retina anterior to the equator, as far as the ora serrata. The direct ophthalmoscope allows visualization to the equator, but not far beyond. The wide stereoscopic view of indirect ophthalmoscopy leads ophthalmologists to prefer this instrument. An interesting but rather unimportant degenerative lesion of the peripheral fundus, *cobblestone degeneration* (Figure 7), is rarely observed by direct ophthalmoscopy and yet is a common observance with the indirect ophthalmoscope. More important are lesions such as lattice degeneration (Figure 116), retinal tears, and vascular lesions. However, the image perceived with the indirect ophthalmoscope is inverted and reversed, and it is difficult to learn to interpolate the image into its actual orientation. The binocular indirect ophthalmoscope has revolutionized both the fundus examination and retinal surgery. Stereopsis, furthermore, provides much greater information about the location and nature of a lesion. Having stated the pros and cons about the more difficult-to-use instrument, the indirect ophthalmoscope, we will hereafter concentrate the discussion on the direct ophthalmoscope, which is more portable and of immense value in itself. The view obtained with the handheld direct ophthalmoscope is comparable to that of the fundus photographs in this book, although its field of view is smaller (Figure 1).

Fundus Photography and Fluorescein Angiography

It is not the intention to describe the technique of photographing the ocular fundus nor to describe in detail the significance of fluorescein angiography. For the beginner, it is important to know something about the technique of obtaining fundus pictures and to learn landmark clues that will tell the approximate location of that portion of the fundus being photographed or examined.

Fundus cameras are bulky and expensive instruments that employ the strobe flash for such instantaneous fundus illumination that motions of the eye become relatively insignificant. The patient and photographer sit at opposite ends of the instrument, as shown in Figure 8. The patient's pupil must be widely dilated. A small fixation light is employed to direct the patient's line of gaze into a field where the lesions to be photographed can be viewed in a direct line with the lens system of the camera. Portable fundus cameras are also available, but the quality of the photographs generally is not competitive.

Under usual circumstances, it is difficult to photograph fundus lesions located anterior to the equator of the eye. The field of the photograph covers 30 to 35 degrees, somewhat wider than that viewed with a direct ophthalmoscope. Recently, a new camera lens system has become available that permits wide-angle fundus photography. However, with wider angles, fundus details are lost. The illustrations in this monograph have been photographed with standard camera lenses and a few (of the macula and nerve head) have been enlarged and cropped.

The appearance of the optic nerve head or the macula immediately provides a landmark that tells the location of the lesion that is illustrated. When these areas are not visible, size and contour of the vascular arcades or the presence of vortex veins (Figure 19) are other indicators that are helpful in ascertaining the actual location from the photograph.

Figure 8. The fundus camera is a large table-mounted instrument. The photographer is shown adjusting a small fixation light to align the patient's eyes in the proper direction of gaze to permit a view of the lesion to be photographed. The pupil must be widely dilated. A strobe flash illuminates the fundus at the instant the picture is taken. Special filters are used with the fundus camera when employed for fluorescein angiography.

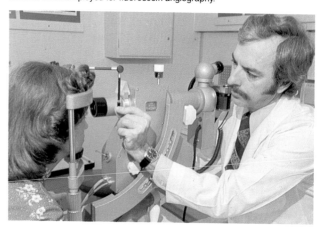

An important technique that has added greatly to the understanding and classification of retinal and choroidal disease has been fluorescein angiography. Following a rapid injection of 5 ml of 10% fluorescein into an antecubital vein, the bolus reaches the central retinal artery in about 8 to 14 seconds, and then passes through the retinal arterioles, capillary bed, and veins in the next four seconds. Actually, the choroidal vasculature fills prior to the retinal vasculature and provides a fluorescent background. The normal retinal pigment epithelium prevents leakage of fluorescein from the choroidal circulation into the pigment epithelium or sensory retina. Normal retinal vessels are impermeable to fluorescein.

Fluorescein dye can, by this procedure, highlight abnormal leakage of choroidal fluid under the pigment epithelium or sensory retina and can expose "window" defects in the pigment epithelium. Neovascular tufts leak fluorescein and thus are easily identified — as in patients with diabetic retinopathy. Usually, papilledema and optic neuritis will cause dilated capillaries on the nerve head surface; these leak fluorescein, and thus cause staining of the nerve head. Furthermore, characteristic helpful fluorescein patterns occur in patients with primary and metastatic choroidal tumors.

Ophthalmoscopy Routine

Approximately 10% of patients studied by fluorescein angiography will be affected with mild nausea or vomiting. The fluorescein dye will discolor the urine and produce a transient jaundiced appearance in the patient. Occasionally, hypotension and anaphylactic shock have been reported—but so infrequently that this ophthalmologic technique remains the most innovative contribution to the diagnosis of retinal and choroidal diseases in recent years.

Examples of single exposures from fluorescein angiograms have been included with this text (Figures 46, 98, 101, 123, 124, 125, and 150). Although fluorescein angiography can be observed through a blue filter inserted in the dial of a direct ophthalmoscope, the rapid sequence of dye passing from the arterial to the venous system and the details of "micropathology" are often missed unless photography is performed and the rapid sequence of photographs is studied using a higher magnification.

It is also well to note that most fundus cameras can provide stereoscopic fundus views, thus simulating the appearance of the fundus as examined with the binocular indirect ophthalmoscope. Such photographs are of great teaching value; however, for obvious reasons, such as cost in reproduction and the need for special viewing systems, they are not included here.

When examining eyegrounds, a systematic procedure should be followed. The room should be darkened but need not be in total darkness. Both patient and examiner should be in comfortable positions (regardless of whether the patient is sitting or supine), and it is best to have a fixation light straight ahead. Without this light, the examination is made more difficult by the patient's eye movements. Touch the patient as little as possible—whether it be with finger, hair, or breath. Be sure to examine the patient's right eye with your right eye and the left eye with your left eye.

Often it is necessary to elevate the patient's upper lid during ophthalmoscopy, but it is more comfortable for the patient and more desirable from the examiner's viewpoint if the lids are not touched except for looking at the lower portions of the fundus when the patient's gaze is directed downward.

The examiner should turn the disc to plus 15 diopters and view the patient's eye from about 12 inches away, looking for an orange ("red") fundus reflex. This plus lens will provide a magnified, fairly clear, red reflex. If dark spots are seen, one should attempt to determine their nature. Any such opacity will be located at the level of the cornea, the lens, or the vitreous. If the opacity is a corneal lesion, it will be recognized by using the ophthalmoscope as a flashlight, casting light on the cornea obliquely. Further, the corneal opacity will be nonmotile except as the eye moves. If the opacity is in the lens, the appearance will depend upon whether the pupil is or is not dilated. Lens opacities are of several types: (1) nuclear sclerosis creates a round, translucent disc appearance, which is most obvious through a wide pupil (Figure 9); (2) cortical lens changes appear as pyramidal or linear markings (Figure 10); and (3) posterior subcapsular and the less commonly noted anterior subcapsular opacities are seen as translucent plaques (Figure 11). Anterior and posterior polar cataracts, which are rare, cause a dense, small, more discrete

Figure 9. Opacities of the cornea, lens, and vitreous obscure good fundus visualization. A nuclear cataract is demonstrated.

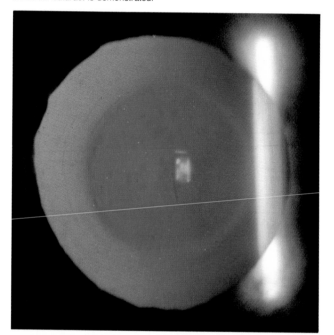

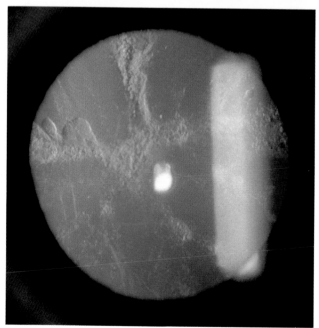

Figure 10. Illustration of *cortical lens opacities* that appear as spokes.

Figure 11. Another common form of immature cataract is a *posteriorly located "plaque"* in direct line with the patient's visual axis. Opacities of the lens are best examined through a widely dilated pupil, with the ophthalmoscope held approximately one foot from the eye and with the lens dial set at " +10 ."

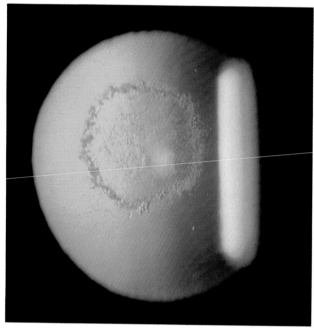

opacity in the center of the pupillary zone.

Vitreous hemorrhages may invade or replace the orange-red reflex; their appearance depends upon their size. When small and diffuse, vitreous hemorrhages are seen as black opacities that move with motion of the eye. If the hemorrhage is recent and is so extensive that fundus examination is precluded, the patient should be put to bed with the head elevated and both eyes patched overnight. Reexamination the next day will be more successful if the vitreous hemorrhage has settled, but many vitreous hemorrhages do not regress that rapidly.

After finding the red reflex, using a high-plus lens, the examiner should ask the patient to look up, down, right, left, and then straight ahead. If there are any "floaters" in the vitreous, these will be seen as the examiner progressively lessens the plus power of the viewing lenses (Figures 12, 13 and 14).

Having thoroughly examined the red reflex, the

examiner should further decrease the plus power by turning the lens dial toward the viewing lens. This will neutralize the patient's refractive error. The ophthalmoscope is now brought closer to the examined eye and fundus details begin to come into view.

Examine the optic disc first, then each of the four "quadrants" (the upper and lower temporal and the upper and lower nasal areas), and finally, the macula. Once the latter has been flooded with light, the patient may become photophobic and less cooperative. For examination of the most peripheral retina, dilate the pupil (page 10), and ask the patient to look as far as possible in the direction of your intended examination (ie, toward the right ear for examining the temporal fundus of the right eye or nasal fundus of the left eye).

With the patient looking straight ahead at some distant target, and the beam directed nasal to the angle of that gaze, the optic nerve is easily seen. In proceeding to examine the fundus, it is important to move the beam and carefully observe the area to each side of the light as well as that portion directly illuminated by the light source. In this manner, dark shadows reveal the presence of hitherto unnoted or unsuspected lesions. When the light is moved from side to side, vague alterations in the smoothness of the fundus can be detected so that, in addition to direct illumination of the lesions, we obtain the advantages of indirect and retroillumination.

When a mass is found during fundus examination and a differential diagnosis between a solid mass and a cyst becomes important, another mode of using the ophthalmoscope may be most helpful. Remove the ophthalmoscope head and attach the transilluminator (commonly used as a handlight). Hold the bulb of the transilluminator against the eye through the eyelid and move the light slightly while viewing the transilluminated pupil; if there are no masses visible, the transilluminated pupil will be illuminated evenly in all quadrants. If any solid masses are present, unless far

posterior, they can usually be clearly seen as black lesions. A positive test response is important; a negative response, however, does not rule out a solid mass.

Now we will return to consideration of the vitreous and will discuss sequential abnormalities in each phase of the fundus examination.

The Vitreous

The vitreous is a gel which normally fills the posterior portion of the eye behind the lens; it constitutes the major portion of the eye's 6.5 ml volume. The vitreous is important ophthalmoscopically because it is frequently the site of both "normal" and abnormal opacities, many of which are evident to the patient. As a rule, the patient with vitreous opacities will complain of seeing spots which he may describe and even diagram as looking like spiders, flies, or threads. True vitreous opacities, as distinguished from retinal lesions, cause motile spots. When the patient has vitreous opacities, he will describe these spots as floating, or as floaters (with some inertia) moving in the direction of the most recent motion of the eye. A lesion of the retina produces a nonmoving blind spot in the visual field that is always at a fixed relationship to the direction of gaze.

The vitreous tends to become more fluid with high myopia or increasing age. It may become detached from contact with the retina so that one may see a dark ring (from its loosened attachment at the optic nerve) floating in front of the red fundus background (Figure 12). The vitreous separation from contact with the retina may cause a transient increase in the quantity of floaters, but it is not a serious occurrence unless the vitreous is abnormally adherent to the peripheral retina – which may then tear and produce a retinal detachment. If the examiner notes a gray or silver elevation above the retinal level, it should be considered a detached retina until proven otherwise (see page 66). Occasionally, one will observe myriads of silvery or golden dots floating in the vitreous, denoting an asteroid hyalosis (Figure 13) of particulate calcium-containing lipid, a form of vitreous degeneration. Synchysis scintillans, or cholesterosis bulbi, occurs in blind or damaged eyes and should not be confused with asteroid hyalosis.

Vitreous hemorrhage is another cause of floating opacities. Large vitreous hemorrhages will appear as floating masses which tend eventually to settle down,

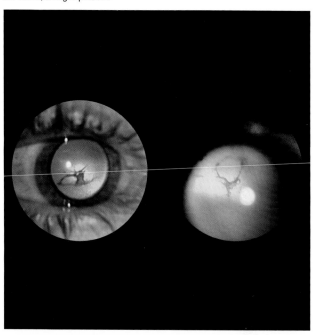

Figure 12. There are many forms of vitreous floaters and opacities. This illustration demonstrates two eyes, each with a *ring-like floater* (often perceived by the patient), constituting a posterior separation of the vitreous from its normal contact with the retina and the optic nerve. Where the vitreous was in contact with the nerve, a ring is present.

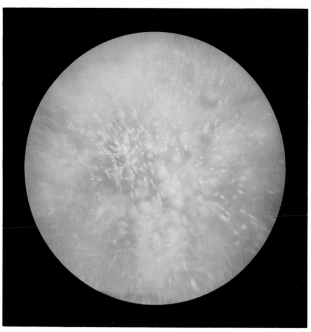

Figure 13. *Asteroid hyalosis* consists of highly refractile calcium-lipid complexes that swirl through the vitreous with movements of the eye.

18

Figure 14. Although the camera is focused at the level of the retina, the blurred image is the result of a diffusion of *inflammatory cells* throughout the vitreous emanating from active chorioretinitis.

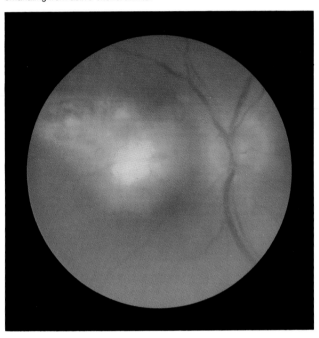

Figure 14. Although the camera is focused at the level of the retina, the blurred image is the result of a diffusion of *inflammatory cells* throughout the vitreous emanating from active chorioretinitis.

particularly if the vitreous is partially liquified. Small hemorrhages will be noted as chains of black "cocci" in the red reflex. Common *muscae volitantes* (the usual cause of subjective floaters, due to usually benign degenerative change in the vitreous) will be noted as small, round, and linear black flecks floating about behind the pupil of the previously moving eye. Worm-like configurations of floaters are common in myopic patients.

Trauma from direct blows to the eye, various retinopathies, and (rarely) inflammations such as severe uveitis are other causes of vitreous hemorrhage. As the vitreous hemorrhage persists, it gradually changes from a red color to a dust-like perfusion of gold clouds and then to a white sheet, and may resorb completely over weeks or months.

Inflammatory lesions within the eye produce a cellular response extending into the vitreous that often cause reduced vision and increased awareness of floaters on the part of the patient. Such cells are seen as a fine gray particulate haze and, if widespread, they may greatly reduce the clarity of fundus detail (Figure 14). Uveitis (page 52) and intraocular nematodes (page 56) are representative causes of inflammatory cells within the vitreous.

The Size and Anatomy of Ophthalmoscopic Landmarks

The "posterior pole" is the portion of the fundus that includes and immediately surrounds the macula. The posterior pole is approximately 3 mm in diameter whereas the macular region *per se* is only slightly larger than the optic nerve head. The fovea, or the center of the macula, is the origin of the sharpest vision and lies just below the horizontal meridian. The fovea is approximately two disc diameters (D.D.s) temporal to the disc (Figure 3). Disc diameters (D.D.s) is a convenient term for measuring the size of a lesion or denoting its site, such as "two D.D.s superotemporal to the disc." *The disc is approximately 1.5 mm in diameter.* One can then describe, for example, a lesion as being one D.D. in size and located approximately two D.D.s superotemporally. This method of measurement facilitates future reexamination of the lesion and assists in determining whether it has changed in size.

When approximate measurements are given, it is assumed that the eye is of normal size (slightly less than 25 mm in anteroposterior dimension) and normal in respect to its refraction (emmetropic). If the eyeball is smaller than normal, it is *hyperopic*, or farsighted; if longer than normal, the eye is *myopic*, or nearsighted. The size relationships as seen with the ophthalmoscope are altered somewhat by the refractive state of the eye. For practical purposes, this does not alter the examiner's estimate of lesion size which is based upon comparison with the diameter of the nerve head.

The optic nerve lies nasal to the center of the globe, and the macula functions as the perimetric, ophthalmoscopic, and anatomic center. The fundus area around the nerve head is referred to as "peripapillary." The nerve lies just below the horizontal meridian and is composed of the retinal nerve fibers. The fibers course to the chiasm and hence to the lateral geniculate body where the fourth order neurons relay the impulses to the occipital cortex. There are approximately one million retinal nerve fibers that converge at the nerve head.

Because there are no rods or cones at the nerve head, their convergence produces a physiological blind spot in the visual field.

Fundus Colors and Contrasts

A knowledge of fundus color pattern and its variations is important. The retina itself is not visible unless it is edematous, at which time it becomes opaque and gray (Figures 65 and 66). The normal orange background color of the fundus is the effect of viewing the retina against the highly vascular choroid from which it is separated by the retinal pigment epithelium. The choroid contains large criss-crossing but nonanastomotic vessels, pigment-containing cells (melanocytes), and a rich capillary layer just beneath the retina.

The retinal pigment epithelium is normally a homogenous pigment layer between the outer (posterior) surface of the retina and the choroid. In some eyes, the choroidal pigmentation may also be uniformly distributed, and in such eyes the fundus background appears uniformly orange (Figures 3 and 21). If the choroidal pigment is unevenly distributed, the fundus appears streaked or tigroid and is referred to as tessellated (Figure 16). This commonly occurs in dark-skinned Caucasians and in non-Caucasians. Such individuals often have a rim of pigment at the margin of the disc. Compare this normal finding with postinflammatory peripapillary pigment of an eye with so-called ocular histoplasmosis (Figure 89). In blondes and redheads, the ocular pigment is minimal, and the fundi appear lightly pigmented with a marked prominence of the choroidal vascular pattern (Figure 17). Also, in lightly pigmented fundi, such as those of very light-skinned blondes and albinos (Figure 18), one may see the four large vortex veins (Figure 19) which constitute the venous cisterns of the choroid. They are not readily observed in more pigmented eyes.

The normal macular area is slightly darker than the remainder of the fundus (see Figures 3 and 20) because there the retinal pigment epithelial cells contain more melanin as well as a yellow pigment that gives origin to the full name *macula lutea* (yellow spot).

With the ophthalmoscope, the macula of young people appears to be encircled by a bright shiny line (Figure 80). If one shifts the ophthalmoscope beam, the fact that a reflex is being observed becomes more obvious. The fovea is visible as a sharp, bright, light spot in the center of the darker macular circle. With age, the foveal reflex disappears or becomes less bright. The fovea is actually a shallow pit in the macula with the foveal reflex appearing as a lighted point at the bottom of the pit.

Observe that the retinal vessels do not extend to the fovea – in fact, their absence at the macula and the surrounding pattern of radially arranged fine vessels helps identify the macula at the time of fundus examination and, of course, in fundus photographs (Figure 20).

The sensory elements responsible for vision include the rods (important mostly for night vision and for perceiving motion) and cones (for day vision, color, and sharp acuity). Remember that these cells are deep to all other cellular components of the retina except for the pigment epithelium. The macular area contains

Figure 15. Another normal fundus is illustrated; this is the left eye and the macula lies to the far right of the picture (compare with Figure 16). Magnification is slightly less in this photograph. Notice the pigmentation at the nasal margin of the nerve head in this dark-skinned Caucasian.

Figure 16. Heavy pigmentation of the choroid is common in brunettes and produces the appearance of a "tigroid" fundus as a result of much choroidal pigment traversed by the choroidal vasculature.

Figure 17. The fundus of a blonde, on the other hand, is characterized by a more diffusely orange color; the choroidal vasculature can be identified (see arrow) where the choroidal pigment is so sparse as to show these vessels against the contrast of the underlying white sclera.

Figure 18. *Albinos* have little or no fundus pigment. This illustration shows normal retinal vasculature overlying a clearly visible choroidal circulation. There are no anastomoses between these two circulations. The macular area. is to the left but is not clearly identifiable.

Figure 19. In this albinotic fundus, a *vortex vein* (cistern of the choroidal venous system) is readily visible. There are four such vortex veins, one in each quadrant of the fundus; when visible they are useful as landmarks for describing the location of fundus abnormalities near the equator of the eye.

Figure 20. The normal macula is shown in the center of the photograph, and the border of the optic nerve head at the far left. Notice the *pigmentation of the macular area* and the fact that the radially arranged fine vessels surrounding the macula do not reach the center (fovea).

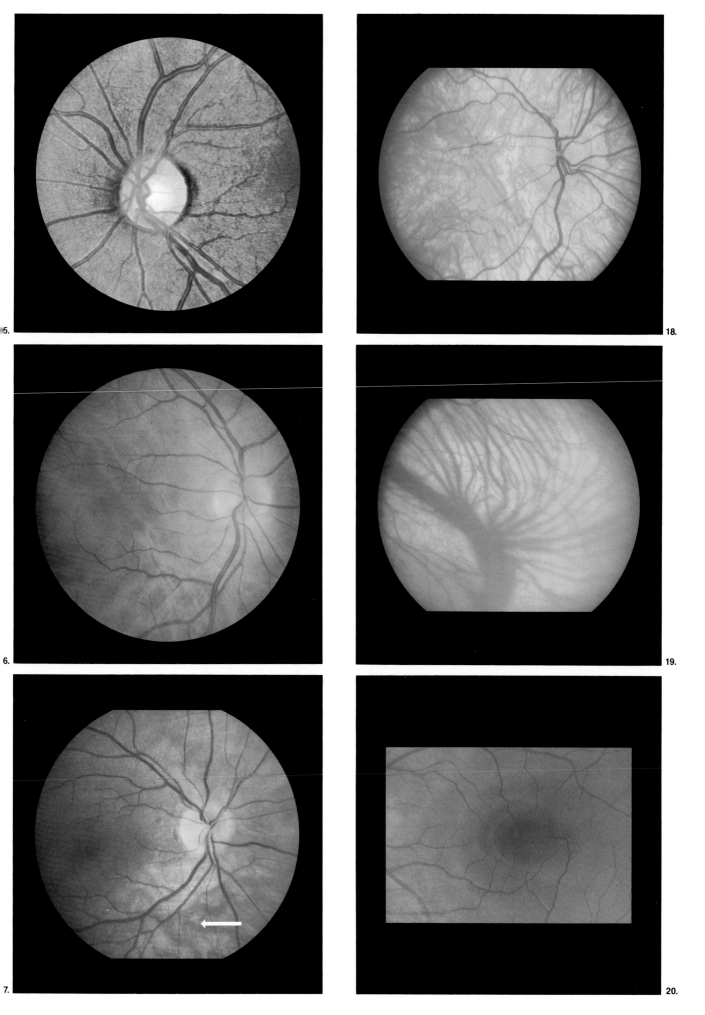

5.

18.

6.

19.

7.

20.

only cones. The outer (distal) portion of the retina receives its nutrients from the adjacent capillary layer (choriocapillaris) of the choroid. Since the thin macula has little more than cones and nerve fibers, the retina at this point receives *all* of its nutrition from the choriocapillaris. Elsewhere the retinal blood vessels cover and obstruct the retinal elements lying directly underneath. An alert person subjected to ophthalmoscopy will comment on the pattern of "veins" that are perceived as an entopic phenomenon: when the patient's eye is examined with an ophthalmoscope, he may note the vascular arcades and the central "avascular" posterior pole. If there is a macular lesion, it will appear as a black central spot.

Deep retinal or choroidal hemorrhages are apt to appear dark gray and may be flat or elevated masses (Figure 61) that can be confused with a malignant melanoma of the choroid (Figure 109). Well-circumscribed, grayish-black, flat lesions are most often benign nevi of the choroid (Figure 104). A dense, black, flat spot usually signifies hypertrophy of the retinal pigment epithelium (benign lesion). When areas of choroiditis heal, they tend to become encircled by retinal pigment which may form a black basketwork over the white scar, but the pigmentation tends to be most concentrated at the margins of the scarring (Figure 87). In patients with myopia, one may see either a fine black or a white crescent at the temporal margins of the disc. In high degrees of myopia, a white conus or crescent may encircle the nerve head (Figure 49).

White tissue has a number of histologic causes. If choroidal tissue is thinned (high myopia) or destroyed (as in choroiditis), the white of the sclera will be seen (Figure 87). Transudates (exudates) as in hypertension and diabetes, or those following the resorption of retinal edema or hemorrhage, are seen as whitish areas that appear "softer" and often smaller than postinflammatory or post-traumatic chorioretinal scars (Figure 62).

Figure 21. Small discrete yellow spots are often seen in the fundus of elderly persons. These *drusen* are most commonly located at the posterior pole and are excrescences of Bruch's membrane which separates the retina and choroid. They have no visual significance other than their tendency to accompany senile forms of macular degeneration.

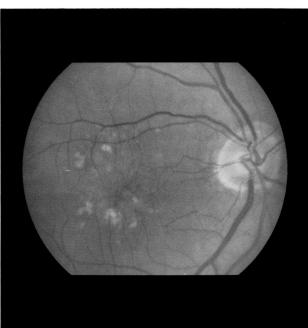

Discrete yellow spots are common findings and should not be confused with exudates. These so-called "drusen" are the result of degenerative changes occurring in a lamina known as *Bruch's membrane* which separates the retina from the choroid. Ophthalmoscopically, drusen appear as small, yellowish, well-circumscribed spots scattered throughout the posterior pole (Figure 21), sometimes outlined by a fine pigment rim. Unlike intraretinal exudates, drusen have a very different appearance when viewed with direct illumination (more yellow) as compared to adjacent light-beam illumination (more pigmented margins and more "translucent"). Fluorescein angiography (Figure 124) shows them to be hyperfluorescent because of the thinning of the overlying retinal pigment epithelium. Drusen produce no visual loss but they may be anlages of senile macular degeneration (see page 73). Inherited (dominant) drusen are discussed elsewhere (see page 81).

The Optic Nerve

The optic nerve contains approximately one million nerve fibers, but it also contains supportive elements. In the normal eye, the optic nerve head is yellowish in color and may have a whitish central excavation (cup) through which pass the central artery and vein. At the depth of the cup, there may be tiny gray dots like pores of a sieve denoting lamina cribrosa that constitutes continuity of scleral tissue bridging the optic nerve's gap in the sclera (see Figure 27). Posterior to this lamina, the nerve fibers acquire myelin sheathing that accounts for the relatively pale color of the central portion of the physiologic cup. Occasionally, myelin sheathing extends anterior to the lamina, reaching a variable distance onto the surface of the retina; this condition should be recognized as a benign congenital abnormality termed *medullated nerve fibers* (Figures 22 and 23). The myelin tissue may cover the retinal vessels, tends to be somewhat striate because it is at the level of the nerve fiber layer, and frays out at that portion most distal from the disc.

Normally the physiologic cup constitutes about 30% or less of the total disc diameter, but there are wide variations of normal optic nerve head appearance (Figures 24, 25, and 26). Since the amount of physiologic cupping of the nerve head is an individual variant genetically determined, the examiner must be aware of certain guidelines to distinguish normal from abnormal. Negroes tend to have broader and deeper physiological cups than do Caucasians. A normal cup, whether deep or shallow, is always associated with a rim of unrecessed, nonatrophic tissue – in particular, at the margin (Figure 26). In distinction, advanced glaucomatous atrophy of the optic nerve head causes a cupping that extends to the very edge of the disc at its temporal margins, creating a sharp border between the nerve tissue and retina (Figure 29). Physiologic cups tend to be bilaterally symmetrical whereas pathological cupping by glaucoma is often asymmetrical.

Figure 22. Occasionally, myelination of the optic nerve does not stop at the lamina cribrosa but extends onto the nerve fibers surrounding the optic disc. This congenital abnormality has no significance but must be recognized as a benign finding.

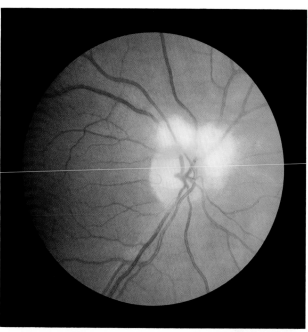

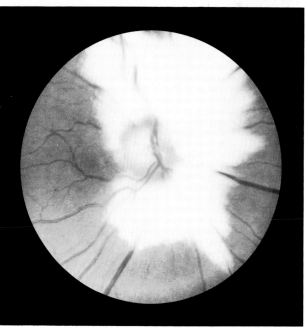

Figure 23. A more extensive myelination of the nerve-fiber layer is shown in this illustration. Notice that the myelination terminates peripherally in a feather-like margin with fine striations resulting from the course of the nerve-fiber layer.

24

Figure 24. A normal optic nerve head is shown. Notice the lighter color within the physiologic cup and the pattern of the vasculature.

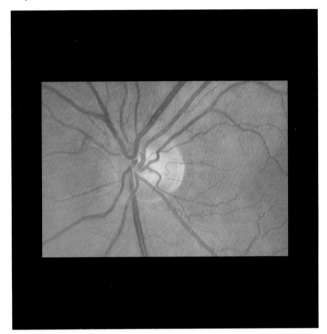

Figure 26. Another normal optic nerve head of a left eye is shown with a sharp-margined, deep physiologic cup having a round contour interrupted only by the presence of the central vessels at its nasal aspect. Compare this cup with the vertically oval cup of an eye with moderately advanced glaucoma as seen in Figure 71 and in Figure 27.

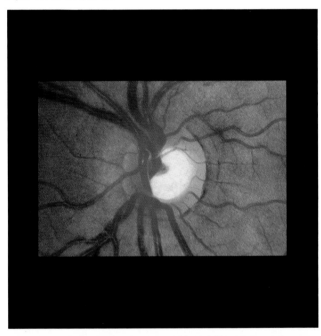

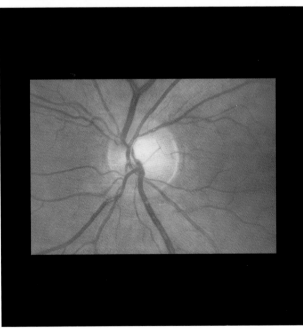

Figure 25. This is a normal optic nerve with broader physiologic cup but a full temporal rim of tissue. The bifurcation pattern of the central retinal artery and vein is unique to each individual.

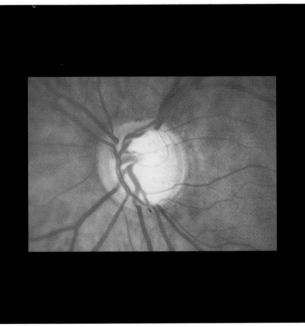

Figure 27. With glaucoma, the physiologic cup broadens first at the superotemporal or inferotemporal location of its rim. This produces a *vertical ovalcy* with *notching* of the cup margin and constitutes one of the earliest signs of *glaucoma*. Such notching can precede demonstrable defects in the visual field.

In ophthalmologic examinations, increasing attention is being given to the appearance of the optic nerve heads in the early diagnosis of glaucoma, but the importance of tonometry and perimetry should not be forgotten as the most important tests for the actual establishment of that diagnosis. A subtle but useful early sign of glaucomatous cupping of the nerve head is the finding of a "notch" in the margin of the cup's contour that causes a vertical distortion in the superotemporal or superonasal portion of the cup (Figure 27). Visual field changes usually correspond well to abnormalities in the optic disc. Notching in the inferotemporal aspect of the cup will correspond to a superonasal visual field defect. As a chronic course of uncontrolled glaucoma gradually ensues, progressive pallor of the nerve head occurs that is initially at its temporal margin (Figure 27). The cup-to-disc ratio (C/D) increases and, as a result, there is displacement of the branches of the central retinal artery and vein toward the nasal aspect of the nerve head ("nasalization") of the vessels (Figures 28 and 29). Far-advanced glaucomatous cupping is characterized by a very pale and markedly excavated optic nerve head. The extent of such cupping, posterior and peripheral to the rim of the nerve head, prevents the examiner from following the course of the vessels from their origin to the nerve head margin (Figure 29).

Glaucoma is only one of many causes of optic atrophy, but the other causes are not associated with increased size of the physiologic cup. In evaluation of both cupping and atrophy, it is important to compare the two nerve heads on the same patient. Generally, both nerve heads tend to show characteristic symmetry, but normal variation can be quite marked if refractive error of one eye greatly differs from the other, as in patients with unilateral high myopia.

Papilledema is a swelling of the optic nerve head, usually related to an increase in the intracranial pres-

Figure 28. The glaucomatous cup of this nerve head constitutes 80% of the horizontal diameter. The cup has deepened to the point that the gray *fenestrations of the lamina cribrosa* have become visible. (This, in itself, is not diagnostic of glaucoma.)

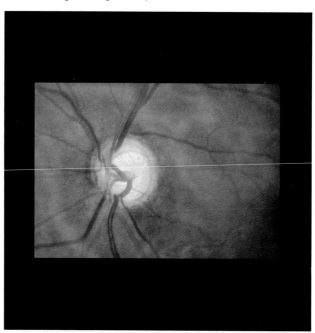

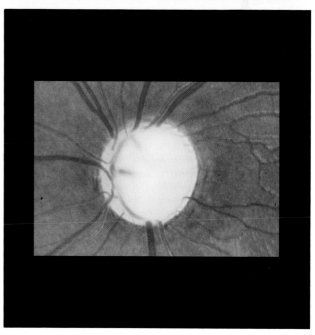

Figure 29. Far-advanced glaucomatous cupping and atrophy are illustrated. Not only does the cup extend across 90% of the disc's diameter, but there is also marked nasal displacement *("nasalization")* of the arteries and veins.

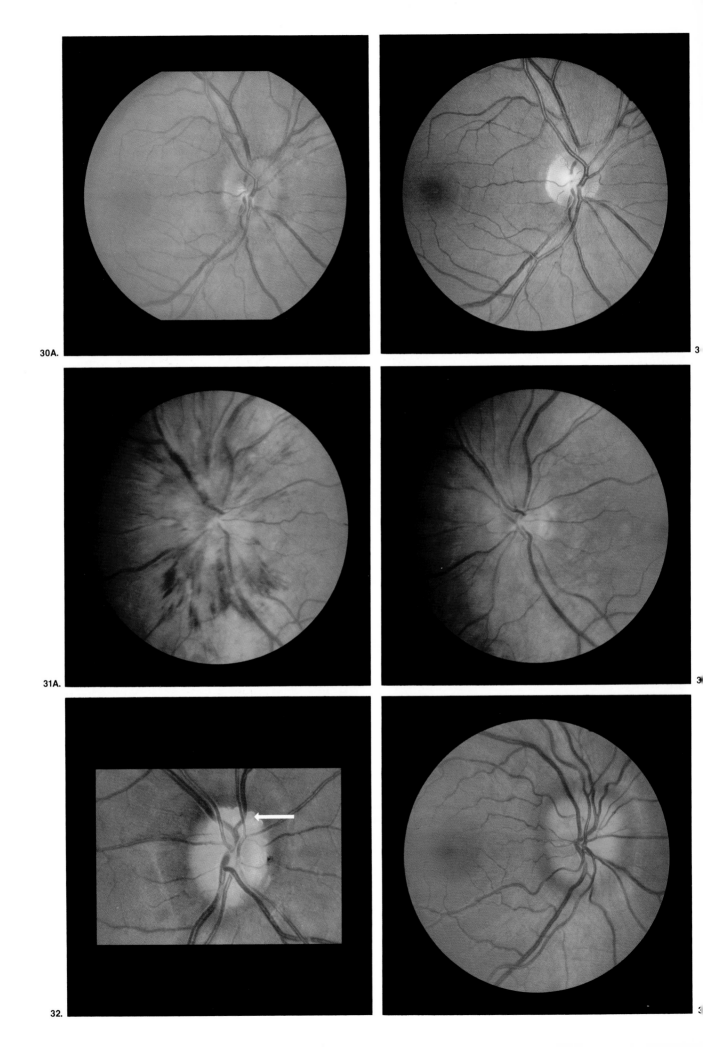

30A.

31A.

32.

sure. However, edema of the nerve head also accompanies a marked reduction in the intraocular pressure (hypotony) and occurs with obstruction of the ocular or orbital venous outflow. Marked elevation in the blood pressure is another cause of disc edema and may exist without elevation of intracranial pressure. In this case, the papilledema is produced by microangiopathy of the nerve head vessels. Notice that in all of these circumstances of nerve head swelling, the term "papilledema" is appropriate, whereas the term "pseudopapilledema" is often used when the nerve heads appear swollen in the absence of elevated intracranial pressure, vascular abnormality, or inflammation (Figures 32, 33 and 34).

Formerly, an elevation of the intracranial pressure was thought to produce papilledema by transmission of the elevated pressure along the potential subdural space that is continuous with the intracranial meninges. It is now believed that papilledema is produced by an obstruction of the venous outflow of the nerve head secondary to an increase of pressure in the cavernous sinus and, hence, ophthalmic vein pressure.

Papilledema is usually associated with normal vision and a slight enlargement of the physiologic blind spot.

Long-standing papilledema may cause secondary optic atrophy and a decrease in vision. Usually no symptoms are associated with papilledema itself. Occasionally, the patient may complain of transient obscurations of vision due to intermittent ischemia of the nerve head. Early papilledema may be difficult to recognize (Figure 30), but advanced papilledema usually presents no diagnostic problem. One of the earliest signs is a loss of the spontaneous venous pulsations in the optic cup. As papilledema progresses, the nerve head swells and elevates. An ophthalmoscopic focus change of three diopters represents an elevation (or excavation) of 1 mm. It is much easier for presbyopic examiners to detect such a change in focus than it is for younger examiners whose power of accommodation automatically compensates for such minimal disparity.

Associated with the swelling of the nerve head is an obliteration of the physiologic cup and blurring of the disc margins. The edema may extend into the surrounding retina, producing a concentric retinal elevation. Flame-shaped hemorrhages and yellow exudates appear near the disc margins as the edema progresses (Figure 31).

In the differential diagnosis of papilledema, hyaline bodies of the nerve head must always be considered. Hyaline bodies (sometimes called "drusen of the nerve head") are usually located anterior to the lamina cribrosa. Although present at birth, these bodies may enlarge during the pubertal growth period. They distort the topography of the nerve head, producing an elevation or multiple elevations that are characteristic (Figure 32). When nodular elevations of the nerve head are not visible, hyaline bodies can simulate the appearance of papilledema due to diffuse blurring of the disc margins and absence of physiological cupping (Figures 33 and 34). Helpful in the proper diagnosis of this entity are the facts that there is no engorgement of the veins, and that other members of the family may be

Figure 30A. *Papilledema* is characterized by blurring of the margins of the optic disc, hyperemia, loss of physiological cupping and fullness of the veins. The vision is usually normal.

Figure 30B. The same optic nerve head one year later, after subsidence of papilledema because of surgical removal of a brain tumor. Slight temporal *optic atrophy* is present.

Figure 31A. Far-advanced papilledema leads to such swelling of the nerve head and peripapillary retina that the disc margins are difficult to identify. Superficial retinal hemorrhages are also present.

Figure 31B. The same nerve head exactly one month later with restoration of a normal A/V ratio and subsidence of the nerve head's swelling as a result of systemic corticosteroid therapy for pseudotumor cerebri.

Figure 32. *Pseudopapilledema* is a blurring of the disc margins not caused by elevated intracranial pressure. The most classic example of pseudopapilledema is that caused by *hyaline bodies of the nerve head.* The arrow indicates the nodular elevation at the superior portion of the disc.

Figure 33. Another example of pseudopapilledema from hyaline bodies of the nerve head.

Figure 34. In this case of hyaline bodies of the nerve head, no nodular elevations are seen, for the bodies lie entirely beneath the nerve fibers. Pseudopapilledema becomes an even more difficult diagnosis with the occasional occurrence of hemorrhage at the disc margin related to the presence of the hyaline bodies. Fluorescein angiography is a useful means of differentiating papilledema from pseudopapilledema.

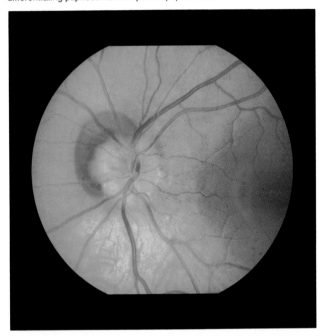

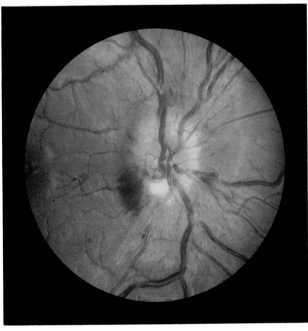

Figure 35. Inflammatory *optic neuritis* may simulate papilledema when it affects the nerve head. Affected patients have profound loss of visual acuity, and frequently there are cells in the vitreous surrounding the disc. Fullness of the veins, blurring of the disc margins, and retinal hemorrhages are characteristic.

similarly affected. Occasionally, hemorrhages occur at the disc margin (Figure 34) and visual field defects may be present.

Patients with marked hyperopia have nerve heads that appear small and often appear slightly elevated. Thus, the diagnosis of early papilledema in a hyperope is somewhat more difficult than in an emmetrope. The absence of disc hyperemia, of peripapillary retinal edema, of hemorrhages, and of venous engorgement are the chief factors that would rule out papilledema. The fluorescein angiogram is of increasingly recognized importance as a diagnostic tool; even with this photographic test, only serial studies and ancillary observations will determine the presence or absence of early papilledema with certainty.

Optic neuritis may involve the entire optic nerve or may selectively affect the retrobulbar portion of the papilla; in the latter circumstance it is frequently confused with papilledema if it merely causes hyperemia and swelling of the nerve head, but if it is further back, no abnormality of the nerve head is visible (retrobulbar neuritis). The various etiologies of optic neuritis include multiple sclerosis, toxic neuropathy, and ischemic processes produced by arteriosclerosis or temporal arteritis. Actually, optic neuritis appears ophthalmoscopically so similar to papilledema that certain differential points must always be kept in mind. Optic neuritis is most frequently unilateral, whereas papilledema tends to be bilateral. Papilledema is usually asymptomatic, whereas optic neuritis often causes pain with ocular motility; it has a profound effect on the visual acuity and produces a central scotoma. An early symptom of optic neuritis is a loss of color vision; specifically, red appears desaturated.

Unilateral optic neuritis in a young person may be the harbinger of a demyelinating disease such as multiple sclerosis. Recent studies have shown that multiple sclerosis patients have a high titre of measles anti-

Figure 36. *Pale papilledema* is never a sign of increased intracranial pressure! In this case it is due to *ischemic optic neuropathy* and in other cases may be caused by temporal arteritis.

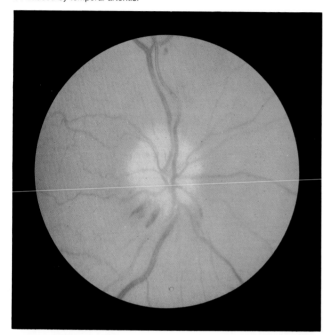

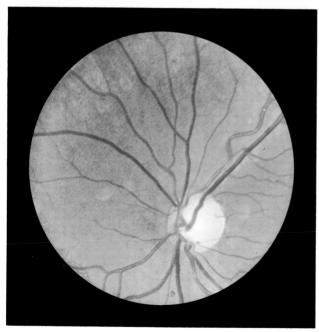

Figure 37. *Primary optic atrophy* is demonstrated by this white nerve head with sharp margins – resulting from a pituitary tumor.

bodies in their sera and cerebrospinal fluid; they also demonstrate a monoclonal immunoglobin-G (IgG) spike. These parameters may prove to identify those patients with optic neuritis who will subsequently develop multiple sclerosis.

The ophthalmoscopic appearance of optic neuritis is that of a hyperemic swollen nerve head with blurred margins and obliteration of the physiologic cup (Figure 35). Venous pulsations are frequently absent as is also true in papilledema. Hemorrhages may occur adjacent to the nerve head. Optic neuritis, being inflammatory, is often associated with floating inflammatory cells in the vitreous anterior to the nerve head. These can be identified as a haze when brought into focus with the ophthalmoscope and can be seen as tiny dots when the posterior portion of the vitreous is examined with the biomicroscope. Such cells usually do not accompany papilledema.

"Pale papilledema" is an ischemic optic neuropathy caused by vascular insufficiency of the nerve head in elderly patients with diffuse vascular disease (Figure 36) or in patients with temporal arteritis. The affected nerve head is swollen but is not hyperemic, as in patients with papilledema and other forms of optic neuritis. The pallor of these swollen discs is important to recognize, for it does not reflect elevated intracranial pressure, and prompt systemic corticosteroid therapy is indicated in an effort to salvage often severely impaired vision in patients with temporal arteritis.

Primary optic atrophy is due to damage to the nerve located posterior to the eye, such as from a pituitary tumor or retrobulbar trauma. There is a gradual whitening of the nerve head resulting from atrophy of the nerve fibers accompanied by a proliferation of glial cells. Primary optic atrophy is characterized by localized or generalized pallor of the nerve head, the margins of which are discrete, and the pattern of the arterioles and veins is undisturbed (Figure 37).

30

Figure 38. *Secondary optic atrophy* as a result of severe inflammatory optic neuritis. Usually there is a slightly more yellow color of the nerve head and *sheathing of the vessels.*

Figure 40. A more widespread colobomatous defect involving choroid and retina in the inferior portion of the fundus is demonstrated in this illustration.

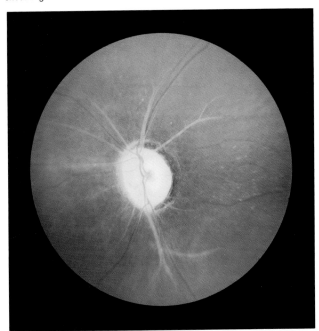

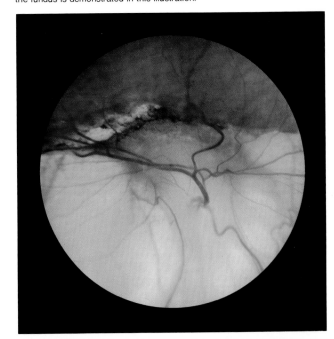

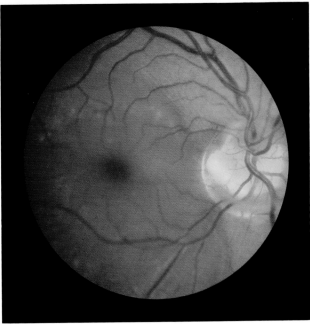

Figure 39. An embryologic defect has resulted in this *coloboma of the optic nerve head* and an optic pit.

Figure 41. *Optic pits* occasionally occur at the margin of an otherwise normal nerve head. They probably represent the mildest form of coloboma and are sometimes associated with serous detachment of the macula, as in this case.

Secondary optic atrophy is the sequelae of long-standing papilledema, optic neuritis, toxic neuropathy, severe retinitis, or ischemia of the optic nerve. The nerve head atrophy may be only sectorial if it is secondary to a localized retinitis. However, remember that some nerve heads have late bifurcation of the papillary arterioles, and in such circumstances there may be fewer large vessels crossing the disc. Such nerve heads, however, have a normal number of very fine vessels on their surface – unless optic atrophy is present. In secondary optic atrophy there may be postinflammatory sheathing of the vessels near the nerve head and disturbance of peripapillary retinal pigment (Figure 38). The color of the nerve head is very pale but not entirely white.

There are numerous congenital anomalies of the optic nerve head. A coloboma of the optic nerve head results from a defective closure of the fetal fistula; it may be confined to the optic nerve head or may include the choroid, retina, iris, and lens (Figures 39 and 40). Depending upon its size and extension, there may be impaired visual acuity and visual field defect. The ophthalmoscopic appearance of the nerve head coloboma is varied, but often the nerve is surrounded by peripapillary atrophy and shows extensive cupping and pallor. The chorioretinal abnormality extends into the inferior portion of the fundus. Probably a mild form of optic nerve coloboma is the congenital optic pit. This lesion is usually located near the disc margin and is often associated with a serous detachment of the macula (Figure 41).

Another congenital variant is *situs inversus* of the vessels, making the right eye's nerve head vascular pattern appear like that of a normal left eye's pattern (Figure 42). The nerve head itself may be congenitally small (Figure 43).

During the early stages of embryonic life, a blood vessel system arises from the optic nerve and extends through the vitreous cavity to the posterior portion of

Figure 42. Another congenital anomaly of the nerve head is *situs inversus* of the origin and preliminary course of the central vessels. This is the left eye, and the macula is located at the extreme right of the photograph.

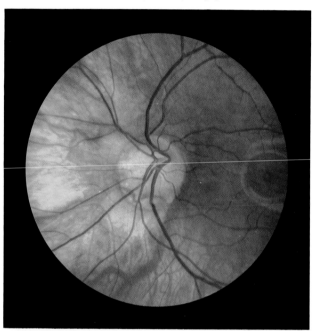

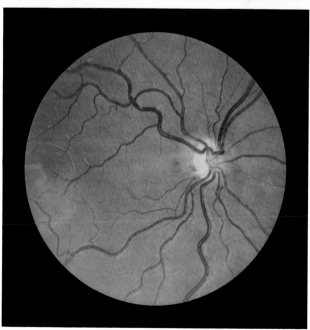

Figure 43. Congenital hypoplasia of the nerve head.

32

Figure 44. Persistence of remnants of the fetal vasculature extending from the optic nerve head to the lens, resulting in a congenital abnormality of the nerve head termed *Bergmeister's papilla.*

Figure 46A. Small, dark, curlicued vascular loops are not neovascular tufts (as occur with diabetes) but are congenital arterial loops without clinical significance.

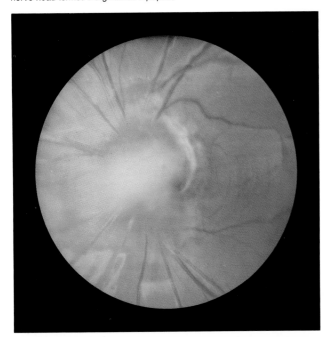

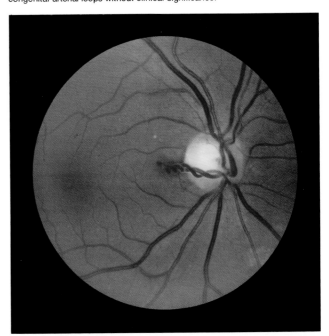

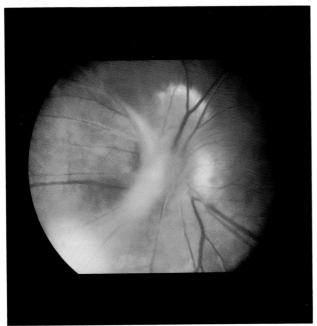

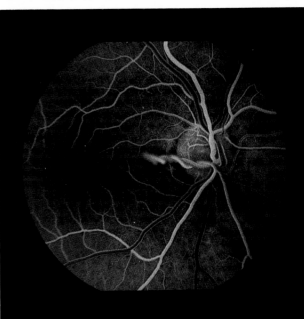

Figure 45. Another example of Bergmeister's papilla.

Figure 46B. That the loop is arterial rather than venous is demonstrated by the fluorescein angiogram with filling of the loop by dye in the arterial phase.

the lens that it enmeshes. This system is known as the *tunica vasculosa lentis* and is of interest only for the residua that may be found on ophthalmoscopic examination: a large, stalk-like vascularized tissue extending into the vitreous cavity from the nerve head, known as Bergmeister's papilla (Figures 44 and 45). Even more common is the finding of an arterial loop that extends from the central portion of the nerve head (Figure 46). The congenital vascular anomalies have a color more suggestive of venous blood, but the fact that they are arterioles is readily demonstrated by fluorescein angiography.

Traumatic damage to the optic nerve head is illustrated by Figure 134.

34

Fundus Changes
Related to Refractive Errors

Myopia is the result of either an eyeball being larger than normal, excessive corneal or lenticular curvature, or an acquired increase in the refractive power of the lens due to cataract. Myopia of more than −7 diopters is invariably the result of increased axial length of the eye; usually beyond this degree of myopia, typical fundus pathology occurs from the excessive elongation of the globe's effect on the vitreous, retina, and choroid. Myopic changes affect the entire eye but are especially significant in the peripheral vitreous, the region of the optic nerve, and the macula.

Nerve head changes are related to an oblique entrance of the optic nerve through the sclera causing a supertraction on the nasal side of the disc with the retina encroaching on the disc's rim. Temporally, there is a white or white-yellow crescent (conus) at the disc margin, due to a pulling away of the retinal pigment layer and increased visibility of the underlying sclera (Figures 47, 48, and 127).

In the patient with a high degree of myopia, the examiner may see large, whitish-yellow areas of circumpapillary atrophy as a result of atrophy of the choroid and stretching of the retina. It is difficult at times to determine where the optic nerve border ends and the area of choroidal atrophy begins (Figure 49).

The stretching of the retina causes cracks in Bruch's membrane and areas of atrophy of the retinal pigment epithelium at the macula (Figure 48). At times, a hemorrhage occurs at the macula, causing a red or black spot at that site (Fuchs' spot) and sudden reduction of central vision (Figure 50).

Figure 47. *Myopia*, when due to increased axial dimension of the eye, is commonly associated with a crescent (arrow) at the temporal margin of the disc. The visibility of the sclera is caused by retraction of the tissue between the nerve-fiber layer and the sclera, choroid and other retinal layers including the pigment epithelium. The earliest form of temporal crescent is shown.

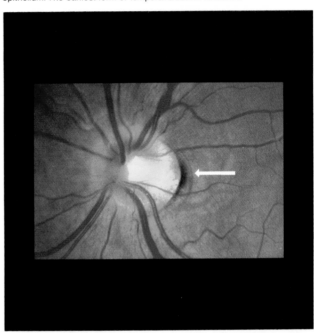

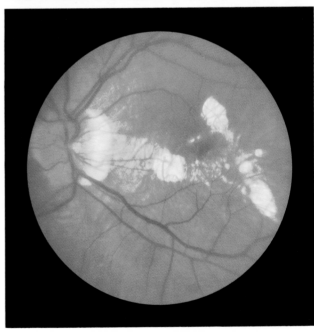

Figure 48. With higher degrees of axial myopia, a temporal crescent is associated with *"lacquer cracks"* and other signs of choroidal atrophy.

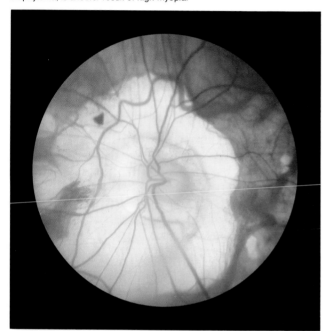

Figure 49. Extensive peripapillary choroidal atrophy and posterior bowing of that portion of the fundus, staphyloma, is another result of high myopia.

Hyperopia has few abnormalities associated with it. Marked factitious hyperopia of approximately 10 diopters occurs when the lens is removed (aphakia). In that circumstance, of course, the globe is of normal anteroposterior dimension. In true hyperopia of +5 diopters or more, the globe is smaller than normal. The only fundus abnormality may be prominence of nerve head tissue that is suggestive of papilledema, as mentioned on page 25.

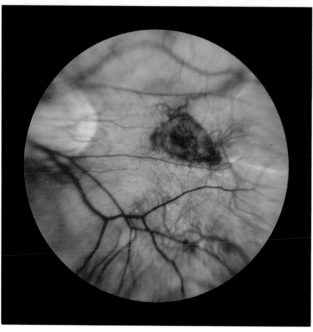

Figure 50. Myopic degeneration occasionally leads to hemorrhage at the macula, the harbinger of permanent impairment of central acuity. This is a *Fuchs' spot.*

Hypertensive and Arteriosclerotic Retinopathy

Ophthalmoscopy is a bit like looking through a keyhole and being rewarded by a view of the occult and beautiful. Study of the "nude" retinal vessels is a very important component of the ophthalmoscopic examination, principally because these vessels are relatively easy to perceive and because they are often affected by systemic disease. Only a few abnormalities of choroidal vessels have diagnostic importance.

The central retinal artery bifurcates to form superior and inferior "papillary" vascular segments, each of which divides to form the temporal and nasal branches that supply the four retinal quadrants. The vessels continue to branch as they extend peripherally. The normal retina (unlike the nerve head) has no collateral circulation and its arterioles do not anastomose. In that the arterial branches lose their muscle fibers and elastic lamina on the retinal side of the lamina cribrosa, *they are arterioles rather than true arteries.* Nevertheless, there are senescent retinal vascular changes that are referred to as "arteriosclerotic."

On ophthalmoscopic examination, the retinal vessels have central reflex stripes, more marked in the arterioles. Pulsation of the central retinal vein is a common and normal finding. The veins are darker and wider than the accompanying arterioles, having a ratio of approximately 3:2 in diameter. The vessels are graceful in their course throughout the fundus, exhibiting gently curving bifurcations. There may be a congenital tortuosity of the vessels, usually affecting primarily the arterioles but sometimes the veins as well (Figure 80). Curving bifurcations are emphasized in that they differ from the acute angled bifurcations observed under circumstances of vessel sclerosis and spasm. Incidentally, the retinal vascular pattern of the nerve head and that extending throughout the retina is as uniquely individualistic as a person's fingerprints, and could (but to our knowledge has not) be used for definitive identification of missing or masquerading persons.

As the vessels pass toward the retinal periphery, the "arteries" (and this word is used by custom and synonymously with "arterioles") and veins cross each other, *with the vein usually passing underneath.* The reverse is less common, but when it does occur, the vein may appear to form a convexity toward the observer as it crosses the artery.

Students of ophthalmoscopy often seek precise statements about what vascular changes constitute diagnostic signs of hypertension and what signs can be considered diagnostic of arteriosclerosis. The response is not easy to provide, for even the experts have trouble with that distinction. First, it is important to understand that arteriosclerosis may be part of a hypertensive process or may be involutional. About 15% of our population has hypertension, and it is remarkable to note how often hypertensive retinopathy is stated to be present when the examiner knows that the diastolic pressure is 90 mm Hg or higher.

Arteriosclerosis of the retinal vessels is signaled by an increase of the light reflex and a reddish-brown discoloration of the arterioles (referred to as the color of copper wire). As this sclerosis of the vessel walls continues, the peripheral arterioles may develop a whitish appearance (referred to as silver wiring). These color changes in the appearance of the retinal arterioles are the result of thickening of the vessel walls. Thus, it is not surprising that where the arterioles cross the veins, compression of the latter will occur. Remember that discoloration of the appearance of the blood column is the result of thickening of the vascular wall, but the wall itself is transparent. At times, the vein will appear to be deflected away by the crossing artery; this is not abnormal, but when the veins narrow and lose their reflex stripes and appear darker on either or both sides of the artery/vein (A/V) crossing, this is significant as a finding in the hypertensive-arteriosclerotic state of the retinal vasculature. Initially, at A/V crossings there is a

Figure 51A. Vascular sclerosis is demonstrated by the segmental increase in light streaking of the arteriole.

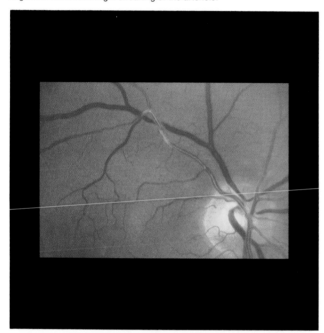

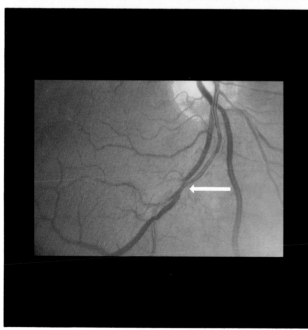

Figure 51B. A/V crossing change (arrow) is shown in the same fundus.

slight deflection in the course of the vein, followed by the development of tapering and constriction of the vein on either side of the crossing arteriole (Figure 51). Eventually, the vein's blood on either side of the arteriole becomes invisible. Although the arteriole and the vein share a common adventitial sheath, the A/V crossing changes are probably not due to traction. Histologic studies suggest that loss of wall transparency associated with periarterial fibrosis produces these ophthalmoscopic A/V crossing changes. Vascular occlusion may occur, followed by neovascular proliferations similar to the more widespread process in diabetic retinopathy (page 47).

Hypertensive retinopathy is characterized in the first stage by focal or diffuse narrowing of the arterioles. These changes may be reversible if secondary to spasm, or permanent if organic changes have occurred in the vessel wall. The degree of the narrowing and the caliber irregularity is usually related to the severity of the diastolic hypertension. The second stage of retinopathy is defined by the presence of arteriolosclerosis copper wiring and A/V crossing changes such as those referred to above (Figure 52). The third stage of retinopathy constitutes the development of retinal hemorrhages and exudates (Figure 53). The fact is that with only arteriosclerosis, many elderly nonhypertensive patients have a few scattered hemorrhages from time to time (often near the optic nerve head or nearby arteriole branches). With hypertension, however, the hemorrhages are flame-shaped, and are located in the superficial nerve-fiber layer of the retina. The appearance of the soft cotton-wool exudates (Figure 62) often occurs rapidly with an acute rise in blood pressure (Figure 55). In severe hypertension, hard exudates identical to those in diabetic patients may be scattered at various locations in the posterior portion of the fundus. Particularly at the macula, they may accrue in quantity to form a star-like configuration (Figure 55).

38

Figure 52. Advanced sclerosis is indicated by the copper-wire color of the arterioles (here associated with hypertension as indicated by the soft exudates). A marked A/V crossing change is noted (arrow).

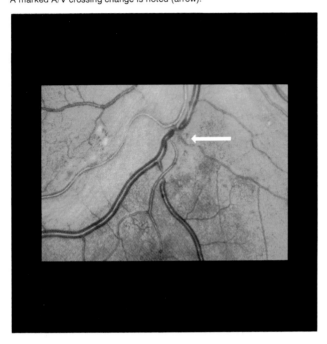

Figure 53. Hypertensive retinopathy with vascular changes, superficial retinal hemorrhage, and macular edema is demonstrated in this 39-year-old patient whose blood pressure is 185/100.

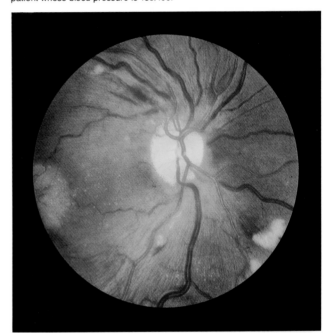

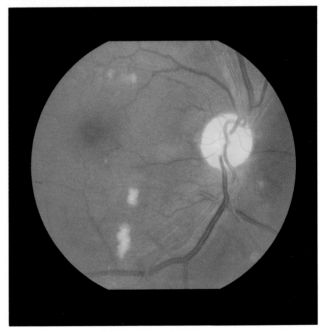

Figure 54. Forty-five-year-old patient has long-standing hypertension with poor control. Notice the soft exudates and A/V crossing change.

The cotton-wool spots and flame-shaped hemorrhages may disappear in four to six weeks. The hard exudates, however, remain for months to years. The most advanced stage of hypertensive retinopathy includes the previously described changes plus papilledema (Figure 56). It is rare to see hypertensive papilledema without the presence of retinal exudates, hemorrhages, and some degree of vasculopathy. The etiology of papilledema accompanying systemic hypertension is usually secondary to an increase in the intracranial pressure; however, some of the affected patients in this category have papilledema resulting from a microangiopathy of the nerve head capillaries. A five-year mortality of patients with papilledema related to hypertension is greater than 90%.

In summary, arteriosclerotic changes include alterations in the vessel wall transparency (as evidenced by abnormal light reflections from the vessel wall) and abnormality of the arteriovenous crossings. Hemorrhages and exudates may occur but are infrequent. Hypertensive retinopathy (commonly associated) may include those changes as well as superficial retinal hemorrhages, cotton-wool spots, and papilledema. Thus, in long-standing hypertension, arteriosclerotic findings are commonly observed; in acute hypertension, reversible vessel spasm accompanies the hemorrhages and soft exudates.

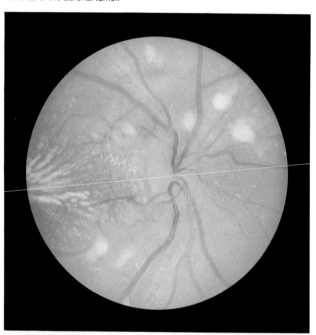

Figure 55. Very acute hypertension in a patient with pheochromocytoma has caused retinal edema, a *star figure at the macula*, and cytoid bodies, but the acuteness of the process is such that copper wiring of the arterioles is not present. This constitutes an acute angiospastic retinopathy. It was reversible with removal of the adrenal tumor.

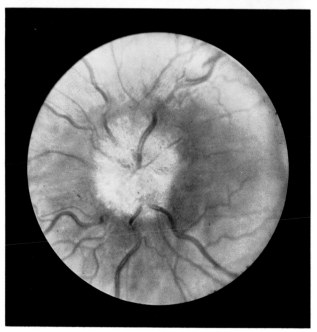

Figure 56. Papilledema resulting from severe hypertension.

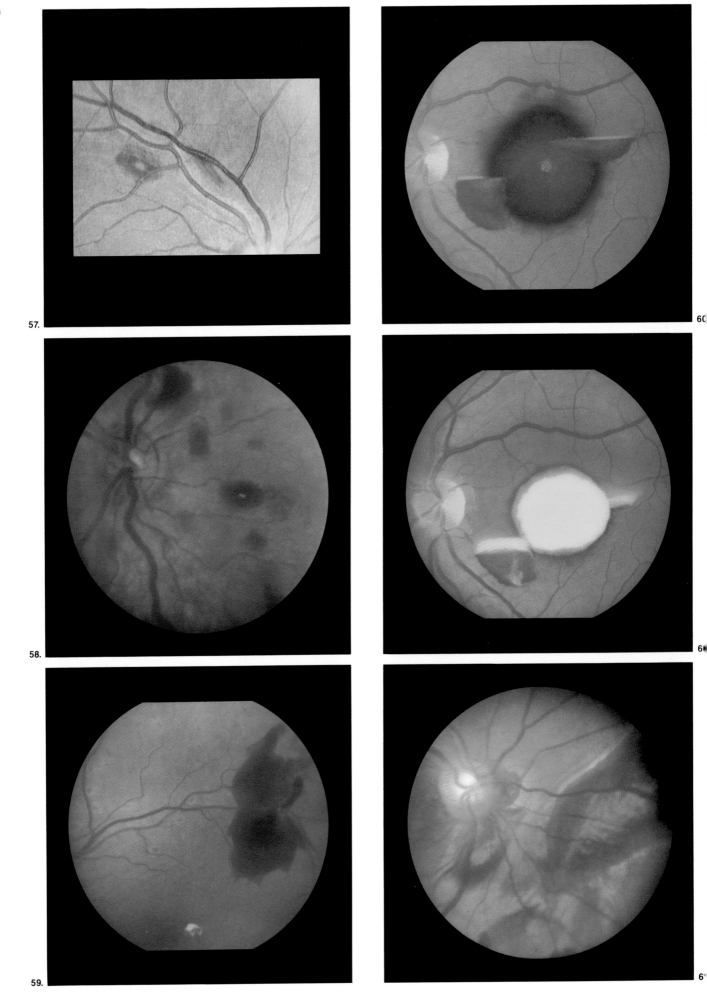

57.

58.

59.

60.

6

6

Retinal Hemorrhages

Superficial retinal hemorrhages are described as *flame-shaped* or *splinter* hemorrhages, depending on their size (Figures 57 and 79). They are located in the superficial nerve fiber layer of the retina and owe their contours to the course of the nerve fibers. These hemorrhages occur in hypertension, anemia, hemoglobinopathies, and other blood dyscrasias.

Dot and *blot* retinal hemorrhages are more deeply located, usually in the outer plexiform layer of the retina (Figure 58). The outer plexiform layer is a potential space for the accumulation of hemorrhages in the presence of venous stasis. Such hemorrhages are small and circular, with discrete borders. Dot and blot hemorrhages occur frequently in patients with diabetes mellitus, carotid occlusive disease, and the hyperviscosity syndrome.

Pale-centered hemorrhages have been referred to as *Roth spots* (although Litton first described them). They are superficial and have a white or yellow center (Figure 57). Roth spots accompany subacute bacterial endocarditis, leukemia, and anemia. Histologically, they constitute a collection of red blood cells surrounding clumped leukocytes.

Normally, the vitreous body is in apposition to the retinal surface. A retinal hemorrhage, however, may extend through the internal limiting membrane of the retina into the potential space between the retina and vitreous, forming a preretinal or subhyaloid hemorrhage (Figure 59). Because of the effect of gravity, the hemorrhage settles and assumes a flat top with a rounded bottom, resembling the profile of a boat (Figure 60). As the hemorrhage is reabsorbed, it leaves a yellow residue that may persist for many months. Preretinal hemorrhages are frequently produced by a sudden increase of intracranial pressure, subarachnoid hemorrhages, forceps deliveries, head trauma, or ruptured neovascular fronds.

Subretinal hemorrhages (between retina and choroid) appear as extremely dark gray or purple homogenous lesions, usually located near the posterior pole. The retinal vessels are seen to course over the surface of the lesion without interruption (Figure 61). This type of hemorrhage occurs following trauma, with bleeding disorders, and is secondary to subretinal neovascular membranes. The hemorrhage must be differentiated from a choroidal melanoma.

Figure 57. *Superficial retinal hemorrhages* are identified by their flame shape. In this illustration, a white-centered hemorrhage is shown: *Roth spot.*

Figure 58. *Dot* and *blot* configuration of retinal hemorrhages indicates intraretinal extravasation. Several hemorrhages in this acutely ill diabetic patient have white centers.

Figure 59. *Preretinal hemorrhages* are easily identified in that they obscure the retinal vasculature.

Figure 60A. Occasionally, deep retinal hemorrhages break through into the potential space between retina and vitreous. The gravitational effect of a preretinal hemorrhage is demonstrated.

Figure 60B. Further resolution of this hemorrhage is observed one month later.

Figure 61. A severe blow to the eye of this patient has led to the occurrence of *subretinal hemorrhage* (dark in color) and minimal superficial hemorrhage (red color).

Retinal Exudates

Cotton-wool exudates are actually microinfarctions of the retinal nerve-fiber layer (Figure 62). These soft or fluffy exudates develop rapidly and may clear in a few weeks. Histologically, the microinfarction demonstrates swollen axon cylinders referred to as *cytoid bodies*. Although ophthalmoscopically the exudate eventually clears, histologically there is permanent evidence of a previous infarction. These soft exudates occur in hypertension, collagen vascular diseases, and diabetes mellitus.

Hard exudates are true exudates that ophthalmoscopically appear refractile and yellowish. They tend to aggregate around the macular area and form faint clusters or sometimes a dense mass with linear markings at the border (Figures 63 and 64). These exudates are composed of serum lipids and fat-laden macrophages that collect in the outer plexiform layer of the retina. The exudates develop slowly and may last months to years, and occur primarily in diabetes mellitus and severe hypertension with nephropathy. Do not confuse exudates with drusen (page 22).

Inflammatory exudates (more properly "infiltrates") are the result of retinal or chorioretinal inflammation. Although the etiology of these inflammations will be discussed with uveitis, there are certain conditions that are more characterized by exudate than by chorioretinal scar. Sarcoidosis is an excellent example of a disorder that may produce not only chorioretinal tissue damage but also retinal exudates – particularly *preretinal exudates* (see page 53).

Figure 62. A magnified view of cytoid bodies demonstrating their "soft" consistency and superficial location in the nerve-fiber layer of the retina. These lesions are *microinfarctions*.

Figure 63. A subsiding post-traumatic star figure at the macula is shown. These exudates may take many months to disappear, in contrast to the rapid clinical disappearance of soft exudates.

Figure 64. Accumulation of lipid exudate at the macula; in this patient, a peripheral vascular abnormality *(Coats' disease)* was present in the same fundus.

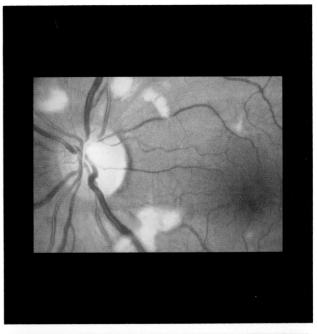

62

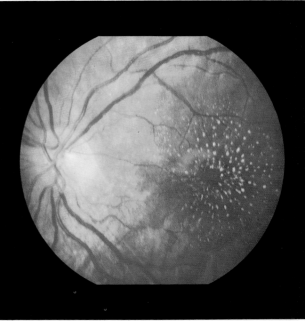

6

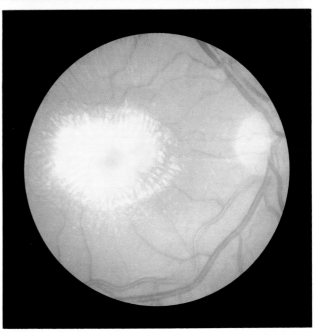

6

Arterial Occlusions

The central retinal artery posterior to the lamina cribrosa is a true artery and is thus subject to atherosclerosis. A central retinal artery occlusion may be produced by a local atherosclerotic lesion or may be secondary to an embolus, and is characterized by a sudden loss of vision, usually profound. Ophthalmoscopically, the entire retina appears to be edematous (gray-white) except for the fovea, which appears cherry-red (Figure 65). At that site, the thin retina is not edematous and permits normal transmission of color from the choroidal circulation. With occlusion, the retinal vessels become attenuated and the disc becomes pale. The presence of a cilioretinal vessel may provide adequate perfusion to maintain retinal function in the macular area (Figure 66). Years later, an old central retinal artery occlusion may revert to an almost normal fundus appearance as the arterioles recanalize, but the vision is not regained and the disc is usually atrophic (Figure 67).

Branch arteriolar occlusions are usually the result of cholesterol or calcium emboli from the carotid arteries or from calcified heart valves. Retinal emboli may produce either a transient or a permanent loss of vision. A transient monocular loss of vision is referred to as *amaurosis fugax* and is produced by a platelet-thrombin aggregate causing transient vascular spasms. However, embolic particles of cholesterol from atheromata of the carotid artery or calcium emboli from calcific heart valves produce ophthalmoscopically visible lesions. These cholesterol emboli have been named for their describer, *Hollenhorst*, and appear as bright, highly refractile plaques which typically lodge at vessel bifurcations (Figure 68). The calcium emboli are white or dull gray and are much less refractile (Figure 69). The platelet-thrombin emboli are probably the most common retinal emboli and yet are the most difficult to visualize or photograph. Since they are soft and pliable, they tend to fragment after rapidly passing through the retinal vessels.

Figure 65. *Central retinal artery occlusion* appears as a diffusely edematous retina with a "cherry red" spot at the macula.

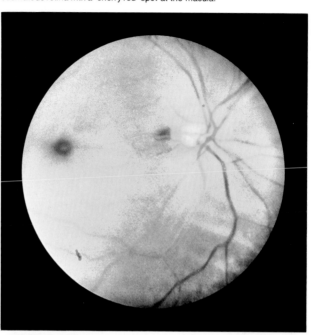

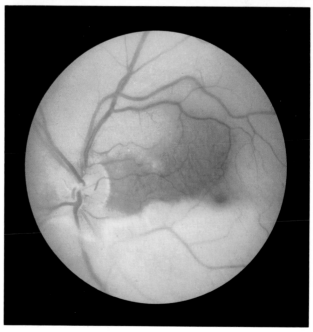

Figure 66. A cilioretinal arteriole from the optic nerve head has led to partial sparing of the retina from an otherwise total ischemia resulting from central retinal artery occlusion. Cilioretinal arterioles derive their blood supply from the posterior ciliary arteries (as does the choroid and optic nerve head) and not from the central retinal artery. About 15% to 20% of normal eyes have cilioretinal vessels.

44

Figure 67. Optic atrophy and a segmental sclerosis of the arteriole branch at the inferior disc margin (arrow) are the only residual signs of a former central retinal artery occlusion. Recanalization of the arterial flow has occurred, but the eye has not regained light perception.

Figure 69. A calcium plaque is seen at the inferonasal margin of the nerve head; peripheral to this location, segmental edema of the retina has occurred. This results in a permanent visual field defect.

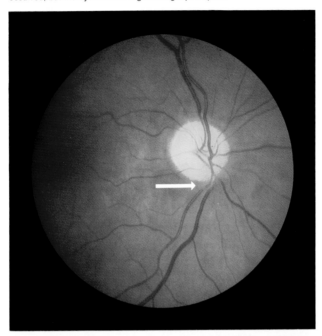

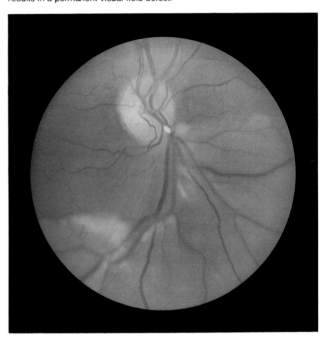

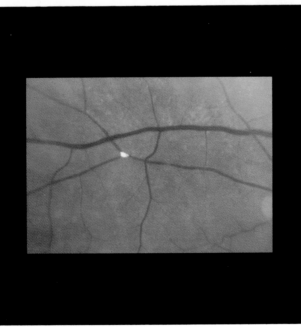

Figure 68. A *Hollenhorst plaque* is seen at the bifurcation of an arteriole. These embolic particles composed of cholesterol derive from the carotid artery system.

Venous Occlusions

The retinal veins are thin-walled and, unlike the arterioles, tend to dilate with increased vascular pressure, forming sausage- or boxcar-shaped segments that are seen with diabetes and the hyperviscosity syndromes (Figure 70). Venous thrombosis is usually secondary to underlying adjacent arterial disease at the nerve head, producing venous compression. Visual loss, however, is not nearly as profound as with arterial occlusions. The ophthalmoscopic appearance is typical: multiple retinal and preretinal hemorrhages surround the optic nerve head (Figures 70, 71, and 72). The veins may appear dilated and the disc edematous, while soft exudates may be present. Recovery of sight may be complete.

Branch vein occlusions usually occur just distal to an A/V crossing. The superior temporal vein is most frequently involved (Figure 73). Ophthalmoscopically, the examiner sees hemorrhages surrounding the vein in the area of occlusion. The visual prognosis is good if the hemorrhages do not extend to the macula with accompanying macular edema.

The medical work-up of vein occlusions includes ruling out chronic simple glaucoma, unsuspected diabetes, and the hyperviscosity syndrome. If macular edema develops, judicious use of photocoagulation near the macular area may be helpful.

Figure 70. The "blood and thunder" appearance of a *central retinal vein occlusion.* There is marked dilatation and tortuosity of the veins, hyperemia of the nerve head, superficial retinal hemorrhages, and soft exudates. Visual acuity is only slightly affected.

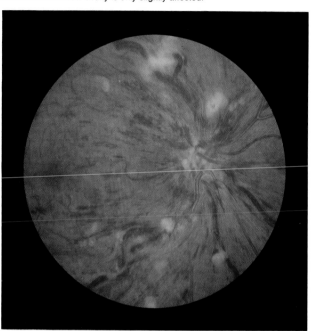

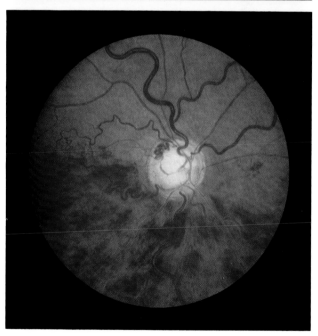

Figure 71. A resolving central retinal vein occlusion present for over six months and now accompanied by early glaucomatous cupping of the disc, as indicated by the *vertical ovalcy* of the cup as well as *temporal pallor.*

Figure 72A. Central retinal vein occlusion with predominance of hemorrhage and little apparent change in the optic nerve head.

Figure 73A. A branch occlusion of the central retinal vein caused by compression of the crossing arteriole.

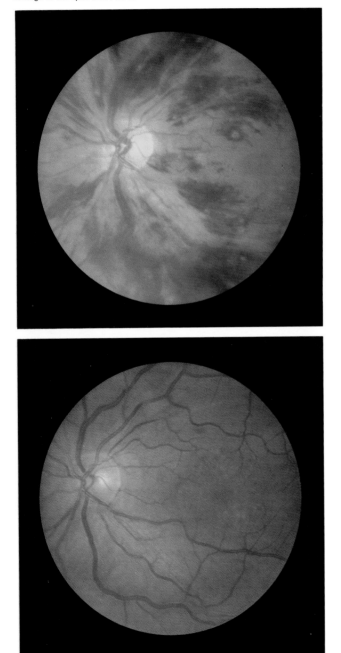

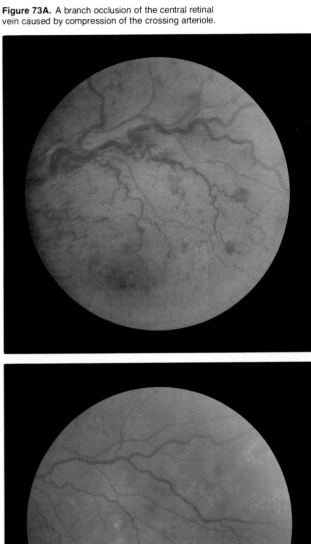

Figure 72B. Same fundus nine months later.

Figure 73B. The same fundus after occlusion of the arteriole and its branches by argon laser therapy. Note the scars from the light coagulation and the subsidence of retinal edema.

Diabetic Retinopathy

Diabetes mellitus has many ocular manifestations. Senile cataracts occur at an earlier age and with greater frequency in diabetic patients than in others. Patients with diabetes may also acquire a transient cataract secondary to retained sugar alcohols in the lens. Sometimes in juvenile diabetic patients, a very rapid snowflake cataract may develop. Neovascularization of the iris (rubeosis iridis) is also a complication of diabetes mellitus and is related to chronic anterior segment ischemia. It is well documented that glaucoma is more common in diabetic patients than in nondiabetic patients.

By far the most serious ocular complication of diabetes mellitus is retinopathy. Although insulin administration can usually control the carbohydrate intolerance, control of the blood sugar levels alone does not prevent the development of vasculopathy. Diabetic vasculopathy is characterized by endothelial hyperplasia and basement membrane thickening of blood vessels throughout the body, including the retinal vessels. The retinal vessels have endothelial cells with pericytes between these cells and their basement membrane. In diabetes mellitus, the pericytes become sparce and the endothelial cells balloon into microaneurysms.

For classification purposes, the retinal manifestations of diabetes can be divided into nonproliferative and proliferative phases. Nonproliferative retinopathy consists of microaneurysms, soft exudates, hard exudates, dot and blot hemorrhages, and edema (Figures 74 and 75). Also included are intraretinal microvascular abnormalities that represent early shunt and collateral vessels. Proliferative retinopathy is the subsequent neovascularization and accompanying fibrous proliferation that may occur at the nerve head, along the vessel arcades and elsewhere on the retinal surface (Figures 76, 77, 78, and 102). What stimulus precipitates the neovascularization is presently unknown, but it is postulated to be hypoxia. Neovascularization may lead to vitreous hemorrhages and retinal detachments.

Figure 74. *Diabetes mellitus* leads to retinopathy in long-standing cases. Tiny *aneurysms* and blot-like hemorrhages occur in the earliest stage.

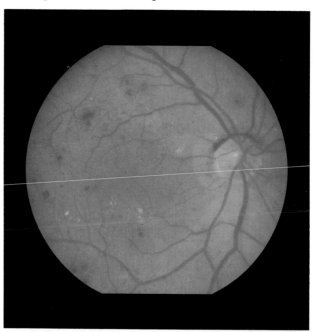

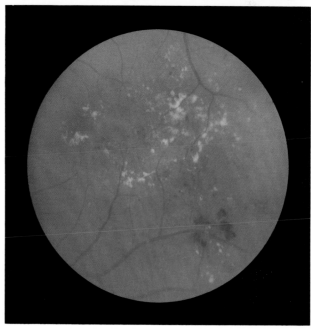

Figure 75. In diabetes, *hard exudates* often predominate, but the aneurysms are always present by this stage and are best demonstrated with fluorescein angiography.

Figure 76. Diabetic retinopathy progresses into the *neovascular stage*. Many new blood vessels are seen at the optic nerve head.

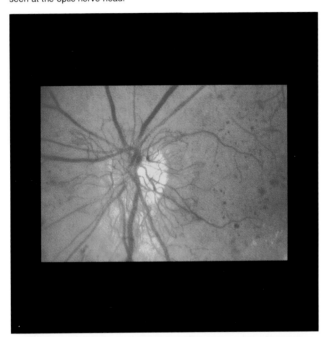

Figure 78. In this diabetic eye, the frond that extended into the vitreous has become ischemic, but the scar tissue is readily visible and the blurred appearance results from diffuse vitreous blood.

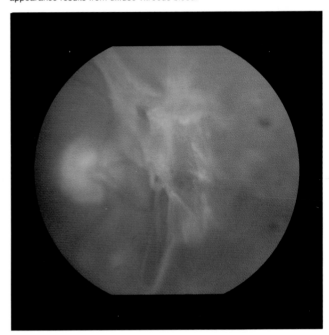

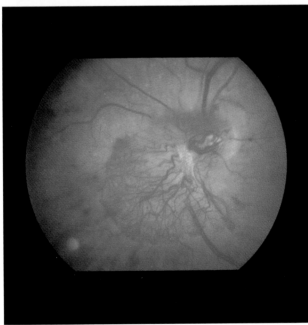

Figure 77. Neovascularization extends from the surface of the retina into the vitreous in the form of large *fronds*. These tend to bleed; the bleeding is then followed by a proliferation of scar tissue, more hemorrhage, and frequently a relentless process leading to blindness.

After ten years of diabetes mellitus, approximately 60% to 70% of diabetic patients show some degree of retinopathy. Fortunately, only about 3% of these patients develop proliferative retinopathy. Proliferative retinopathy is rare in the very young and the very old. Prior to fifteen years ago, pituitary ablation was the only surgical method for attempted control of proliferative retinopathy. It was thought that destroying growth-hormone-producing cells would retard or reverse the neovascularization. Although moderately successful, pituitary ablation was fraught with complications. For the past two decades, photocoagulation with the xenon arc or laser have become the most common mode of treatment of diabetic retinopathy, but reliable data regarding the efficacy of such light coagulation remain to be reported conclusively.

Blood Disorders

The color of the ocular fundus is due to the pigmentation and blood flow of the retina and choroid. Alterations in the blood volume such as in anemia, polycythemia, and hyperviscosity can produce distinctive ophthalmoscopic abnormalities. Likewise, leukemic infiltrates and abnormally sickled red blood cells can produce ocular vessel abnormalities and hemorrhages.

ANEMIA

The ophthalmoscopic findings of anemia are usually directly proportional to the hemoglobin level. Increasing paleness of the fundus parallels reduction of the hematocrit. When the hemoglobin is less than 8 gm%, retinal hemorrhages often occur. The development of retinal hemorrhages itself is potentiated by a concurrent decrease in circulating platelets. A combination of anemia and thrombocytopenia, with platelet counts below 50,000/mm, predisposes to retinal hemorrhages. The hemorrhages seen in anemia are superficial and flame-shaped. This overall fundus appearance is rather pale because of decreased amounts of perfusing hemoglobin. Frequently, one sees soft cotton-wool exudates as a result of infarction of the nerve-fiber layer. If the anemia develops very rapidly, as in a massive gastrointestinal hemorrhage, one may actually observe spasm of the central retinal artery and its branches. If exsanguination is extremely severe, infarction of the retina may occur as a result of central retinal artery occlusion. However, if the anemia develops slowly over a long period of time, the optic nerve head may slowly develop a pale appearance secondary to chronic ischemia that eventually produces a secondary optic atrophy.

LEUKEMIA

The ocular manifestations of leukemia are primarily located in the retina and choroid. Retinal hemorrhages and choroidal infiltrates are very common in leukemia (especially in the acute forms) and are related to the white blood cell count, hemoglobin level, and platelet titre. Since over half of the patients presenting with acute leukemia are anemic and thrombocytopenic, it is not unusual that retinal hemorrhages are common ophthalmoscopic findings. The hemorrhages are usually superficial (flame-shaped), similar to those of hypertension and anemia. Occasionally, pale-centered hemorrhages are noted. Histologically, these pale-centered hemorrhages in leukemia patients are composed of red cells surrounding a core of leukocytes. If the leukemia is severe, preretinal hemorrhages may ensue. Extreme elevation of the white count can lead to occlusion of peripheral retinal arterioles and subsequent neovascularization of the retinal periphery. Papilledema also occurs; such unilateral nerve head swelling is usually secondary to abnormal leukocytes that obstruct the venous outflow of the nerve head. True bilateral papilledema is secondary to leukemic involvement of the central nervous system.

HYPERVISCOSITY SYNDROMES

Hyperviscosity syndromes are caused by an increase in serum proteins and cellular elements. Normally, the serum viscosity is approximately 1.2 to 1.6 times that of water. The conditions that produce hyperviscosity include Waldenström's macroglobulinemia, multiple myeloma, cryoglobulinemia, polycythemia, and leukemia. Of these, Waldenström's macroglobulinemia produces the greatest degree of viscosity and the most severe clinical manifestations. In macroglobulinemia, there is an increase in the IgM immunoprotein. The molecular weight of IgM is approximately one million and the protein is almost entirely intravascular. These factors contribute to the extreme hyperviscosity of macroglobulinemia. Viscosity syndromes can produce cerebrovascular accidents, congestive heart failure, and diffuse bleeding from mucous membranes.

The vascular changes usually become apparent when

50

the viscosity reaches approximately five times that of water. The retinal blood vessels, especially the veins, become extremely dilated; retinal hemorrhages occur, and the fundus may simulate the appearance of a central retinal vein thrombosis (Figure 79). Marked dilatation of the veins leads to boxcar or sausage-chain segmentations. The hyperviscosity syndrome secondary to increased serum proteins is best treated by plasmaphoresis. The fundus appearance then returns to normal, and there is a return of normal vision as the associated macular edema subsides.

HEMOGLOBINOPATHIES

The hemoglobinopathies are a group of disorders characterized by abnormal molecular hemoglobin proteins; they may produce characteristic ocular lesions. Sickle cell anemia (Hgb S-S) occurs in about 0.4% of the black population, whereas sickle cell trait (S-A) occurs in approximately 10% of that population. Other types of hemoglobinopathies that may affect the eye include sickle cell thalassemia (S-thal) and sickle cell hemoglobin C disease (S-C).

The ocular manifestations of these hemoglobinopathies are related to the number of sickled red cells, the hematocrit, and the serum viscosity. Vascular changes (some transient) can be found in the conjunctiva, retina, and choroid. Patients with sickle cell disease have a variable number of sickled cells that may sludge conjunctival vascular flow, producing short comma-shaped segmentations of the capillaries that are pathognomonic. Because of the sickled cells and increased viscosity, there is usually an increased tortuosity of the retinal vasculature (Figure 81). The peripheral retinal blood vessels sometimes become occluded, especially with the S-C and S-thal forms. Occlusion is the first step in a sequence of events that may eventually lead to recurrent vitreous hemorrhages and retinal detachment. After the peripheral blood vessels occlude, local A/V

Figure 79A. Marked engorgement of the veins and superficial retinal hemorrhages in a patient with Waldenström's macroglobulinemia.

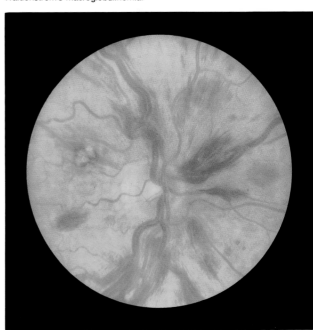

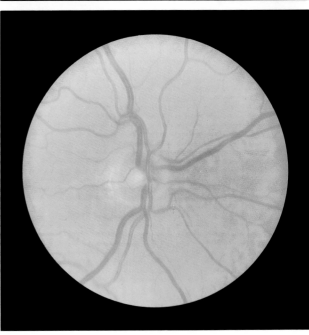

Figure 79B. The same eye several months later following treatment by plasmaphoresis.

Figure 80. A normal fundus of a young Negro
patient showing congenital *tortuosity of the
vasculature* and the typical silk-like light reflexes
on the fundus that are characteristic of youth.

Figure 82. A typical *sea-fan* vascular proliferation in
the peripheral retina of a patient with sickle cell-C disease.

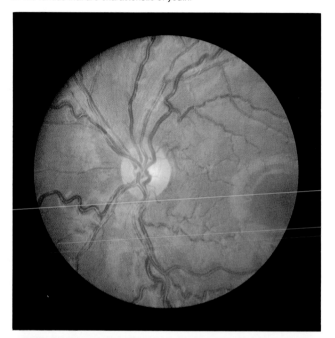

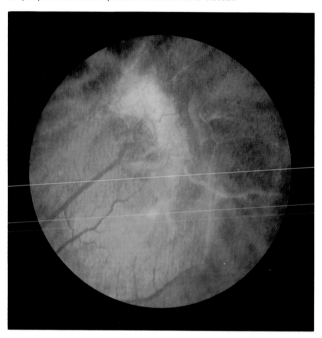

shunts develop; this is followed by the appearance of neovascularization extending in a sea-fan distribution toward the ora serrata (Figure 82). These neovascular tufts are fragile and some of them hemorrhage into the vitreous. This peripheral occlusive process is seen more commonly in S-C disease than it is in S-S disease, probably because in S-C disease the serum hemoglobin (and hence viscosity) is higher than in S-S disease – thus promoting peripheral arteriolar occlusion. Angioid streaks (page 87) are seen in approximately 5% of clinically significant cases of sickle cell disease.

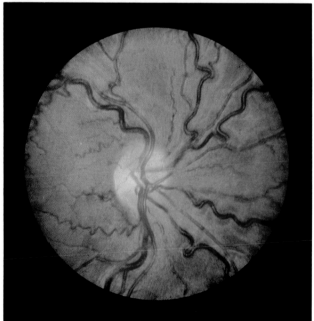

Figure 81. Fundus of a Negro patient showing
marked vascular tortuosity. In this case, the patient
has *sickle cell anemia.* Vascular tortuosity alone
is not sufficient for a diagnosis but leads to a
suspicion of sickle cell disease.

Inflammations (Retinitis and Choroiditis)

This group of inflammations may be acute or chronic. Some inflammatory conditions have a characteristic appearance and others are nonspecific. Some forms of retinitis and choroiditis are merely inflammatory infiltrates; others are granulomatous reactions leading to neovascular membranes and retinal pigmentary alterations. Most of these inflammations are acquired, although diseases such as rubella, syphilis, and toxoplasmosis may be the result of intrauterine infection.

SARCOIDOSIS

Sarcoidosis is a disease of unknown etiology with noncaseating granulomatous involvement of multiple tissues and organs. Sarcoidosis is a disease primarily of young people; over 70% of affected individuals are under 40 years of age. Males and females are affected equally. The tissues involved most frequently are the lungs, hilar nodes, peripheral lymph nodes, liver, skin, and bone. However, the nervous system is rarely involved. Other unusual manifestations of sarcoidosis include allergy to many skin tests; over 60% of patients with sarcoid do not respond to tuberculin skin testing. There is often a nonspecific elevation of the gamma globulins and a significant hypercalcemia. Intrathoracic involvement may range from bilateral hilar adenopathy to diffuse pulmonary infiltration.

Tissue extracts from the lymph nodes of sarcoid patients, when injected in others with sarcoidosis, produce a cutaneous response. This test, the Kveim-Siltzbach reaction, is positive in over 80% of patients having the disease.

Ocular involvement has been noted in approximately 25% of these affected patients. The ocular and periorbital involvement in sarcoid is diffuse. Cutaneous lid granulomatas are not infrequent and may be quite disfiguring. Conjunctival nodules may serve as a source of biopsy material for diagnostic purposes; the lacrimal and the parotid glands also may be involved. Extensive

Figure 83. Exudates along the course of fundus vessels are shown in this patient with *sarcoidosis*.

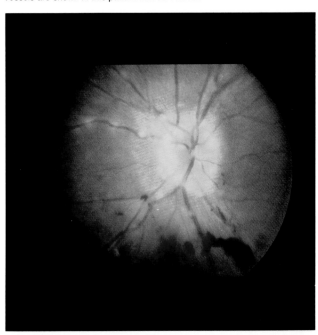

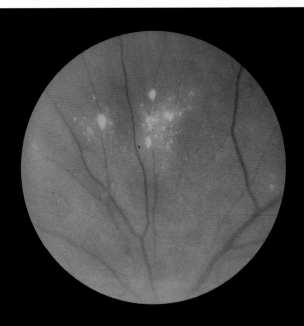

Figure 84. *Candle-wax dripping* is the description applied to these preretinal exudates in another patient with sarcoidosis.

Figure 85. The typical appearance of a healed scar from *toxoplasma chorioretinitis*.

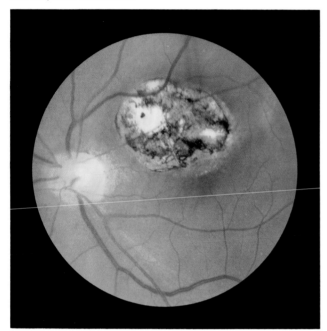

lacrimal involvement may produce hypolacrimation and secondary keratitis sicca. Iritis is both the most common ocular manifestation and the usual presenting ocular symptom of sarcoid, characterized by a granulomatous reaction in the anterior chamber. Slit-lamp examination may reveal mutton-fat or greasy keratic precipitates (KPs) on the endothelium of the cornea. Sarcoid nodules are sometimes noted on the iris itself. The vitreous may demonstrate a secondary cellular response and there may even be actual granulomata in the vitreous body. Inflammatory exudates also may be found in the choroid and retina and on the optic nerve head. Frequently, the blood vessels, especially the retinal veins, demonstrate sheathing, which is a perivascular response to inflammation. Sometimes the vasculitis is the most outstanding ophthalmoscopic feature, with widespread vascular occlusions and hemorrhages, as well as vascular sheathing (Figure 83). In the vicinity of the sheathing, *preretinal* inflammatory exudates re-

ferred to as "candle-wax drippings" may be detected (Figure 84). These are noteworthy because when present they are almost diagnostic, and they portend central nervous system involvement. Additionally, granulomata of the nerve head may simulate papilledema. True papilledema may be observed with central nervous system involvement, which causes a secondary increase in the intracranial pressure. Ocular sarcoid may be treated by topical, subconjunctival, or systemic corticosteroids.

Although the 10-year survival rate with sarcoid is greater than 85%, some patients suffer severe complications. The sarcoid lesions heal by fibrosis and scarring of the organs involved, including the ocular tissues – although exudates themselves may disappear without residua.

TOXOPLASMOSIS
Toxoplasmosis is the most common cause of chorioretinitis in the United States. The toxoplasma organism is an obligate intracellular parasite carried by animals. The cat appears to be a definitive host and transmits the infectious oocyst to man. It is also known that human infection may be either congenital or acquired. Acute systemic toxoplasmosis produces a viral-like syndrome with fever and lymphadenopathy.

The ocular inflammation is characterized by an acute chorioretinitis beginning initially with retinal involvement. The early lesions appear yellow-white, with a marked inflammatory reaction in the adjacent vitreous (Figure 14). These lesions heal, forming markedly pigmented chorioretinal scars (Figure 85). Subsequent lesions may develop adjacent to the older lesions, again appearing creamy white or yellow-white with an overlying cellular reaction in the vitreous (Figure 86). The toxoplasma organism becomes a dormant encapsulated cyst in the retinal tissue. If there is an alteration in, or breakdown of, the local tissue immunity, the orga-

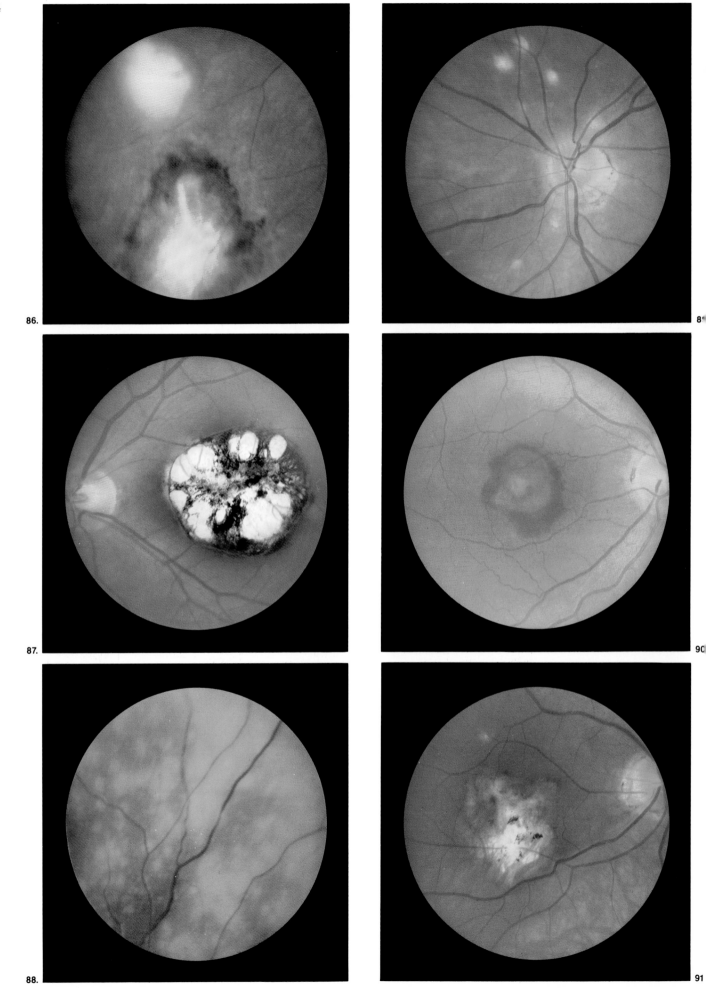

54

86.

8

87.

90

88.

91

nism will immediately spread to adjacent retinal tissue.

Congenital infection has a predilection for involving the macula and is acquired by the fetus from the mother via transplacental spread (Figure 87). If the organism is transmitted to the fetus during the first trimester, the ocular and cerebral complications usually are severe. Fortunately, transmission of the organism during the first trimester is unusual. It is during the last trimester that the organism is most frequently transmitted and at this time the morbidity is less.

There are multiple serologic tests that corroborate the diagnosis of toxoplasmosis. A high percentage of the United States population has a positive antibody titre to the toxoplasma organism. The classic treatment of ocular toxoplasmosis consists of sulfanilamides, pyrimethamine, and corticosteroids.

CYTOMEGALIC INCLUSION RETINITIS

The cytomegaloviruses are DNA viruses belonging to the same general group as herpes simplex. Although exposure to this virus is widespread, as evidenced by the presence of complement-fixing antibodies in a high percentage of adults over the age of 35, the virus rarely produces a clinically recognized disease. When it affects children, usually in the congenital form, it is manifested by prematurity, hematologic reticuloendothelial changes, cerebral calcifications, and chorioretinitis. Although the disease is rarely encountered in healthy

Figure 86. Inferiorly located is a healed scar of toxoplasma chorioretinitis. Superiorly, an active lesion without pigmentation is seen.

Figure 87. Congenital toxoplasmosis, when it affects the eye in utero, has a predilection for destruction of the macula, as shown in this patient.

Figure 88. *Cytomegalic virus* can produce a rampant retinitis.

Figure 89. Common in many parts of the country is the so-called *ocular histoplasmosis syndrome*, characterized by peripapillary scarring and punctate, well-circumscribed spots scattered throughout the fundus.

Figure 90. *Hemorrhagic macular degeneration* is a common accompaniment of the ocular histoplasmosis syndrome.

Figure 91. The late sequelae of macular hemorrhage have led to scarring and permanent loss of central acuity in this patient with ocular histoplasmosis.

adults, it may present as an interstitial pneumonitis or nonspecific viral syndrome. Patients with suppression of their immunologic surveillance secondary to malignancies, lymphomas, or leukemias are prone to cytomegalovirus infections. Also, patients on prolonged immunosuppressive therapy following renal transplantation have a high frequency of cytomegalic infections.

Ocular involvement of cytomegalovirus was initially observed in infants. The virus has been recovered from the anterior chamber of these patients. The characteristic ophthalmoscopic picture consists of white dots, scattered near sheathed vessels. Eventually, the patches of retinitis become confluent (Figure 88) and vascular occlusions may occur. Subsequently, extensive areas of retinal pigment epithelial atrophy are covered by retinal fibrosis. The virus produces most of its damage in the retina; Bruch's membrane apparently protects the choroid.

There is no effective treatment for the cytomegalic virus. Gamma globulin, interferon inducers, and even transfer factor have all been used unsuccessfully.

HISTOPLASMOSIS

The so-called ocular histoplasmosis syndrome is characterized by peripapillary scarring associated with peripheral small discrete chorioretinal scars (Figure 89). Occasionally, the observer will find a lesion or two in its active phase with minimal surrounding edema and inflammatory response. The macular area is frequently involved with recurrent hemorrhages (Figure 90) and an end stage of chorioretinal scarring (Figure 91). The constellation of macular lesions, peripheral punctate scars, and peripapillary scarring is characteristic of this syndrome.

Only rarely has the histoplasma organism been identified in the eye with any certainty. The ocular reaction is thought to be a hypersensitivity or autoimmune response to systemic histoplasmosis. Patients with this

56

ophthalmologic constellation frequently have a positive serologic and skin reaction to histoplasma antigen. There is no known systemic treatment for ocular histoplasmosis; however, the neovascular membranes are sometimes amenable to photocoagulation treatment. When macular involvement occurs, the prognosis for long-term maintenance of good central vision is poor. Systemic corticosteroids are often used but without demonstrable benefit in carefully analyzed case studies.

SYPHILIS

The ocular manifestations of luetic infections consist of interstitial keratitis, pupillary abnormalities, readily dislocated lenses, optic atrophy, and chorioretinitis. Although the resultant chorioretinal scarring is not diagnostic, luetic chorioretinal damage tends to be widespread throughout both fundi and is associated with retinal pigment clumping similar to that of retinitis pigmentosa (Figure 92). Luetic chorioretinitis is sometimes associated with a positive serologic reaction, especially a positive FTA-ABS test. Patients with a positive serologic reaction should be treated with an appropriate and adequate course of antibiotics if this has not been done previously. Syphilis has many forms, and both congenital and acquired luetic infections can affect the ocular fundus.

INTRAOCULAR NEMATODE

Children have the greatest likelihood of ingesting the ova of nematodes, especially *Toxocara canis*. The ova from mature worms are passed in the feces of the host animal, and when these ova are ingested by children, they hatch in the small intestine. The larvae then migrate via the blood and lymph channels, reaching the liver, lungs, and other organs where they produce a granulomatous reaction. In the human, these organisms never mature. The blood-borne larva reaches the eye, where it may produce an intraocular granuloma or an

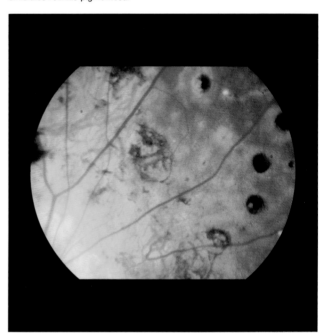

Figure 92. *Congenital syphilis* produces a diffuse chorioretinal postinflammatory scarring that often simulates retinitis pigmentosa.

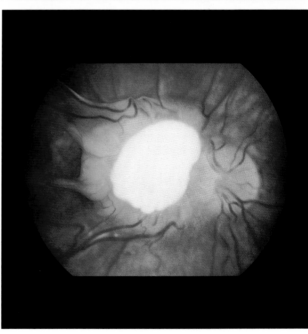

Figure 93. The nematode, *Toxocara cana*, enters the eye in childhood; the worm dies, leaving a gliotic mass.

Figure 94. Another case of *Toxocara cana*: a diffuse scarring from preretinal inflammation has led to retinal traction.

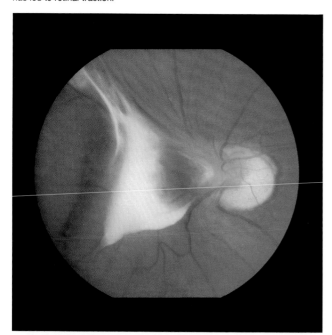

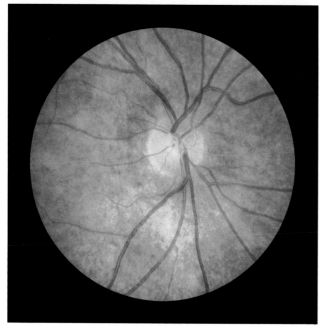

Figure 95. *Congenital rubella* leads to the *"salt and pepper"* chorioretinal scarring illustrated by this fundus.

endophthalmitis with a severe vitreous reaction. Migration of the larva may produce ophthalmoscopically visible tracks across the retinal surface; inflammation is minimal or absent until the larva dies. The organism then produces a retinal and subretinal reaction which eventually scars with glial proliferation, either at the posterior pole (Figure 93) or in the retinal periphery. The retina may be thrown into folds (Figure 94) or may actually detach. The white, elevated, cocoon-like scar is quite characteristic, although it may simulate a retinoblastoma. It is always unilateral and is not multifocal.

CONGENITAL OCULAR RUBELLA SYNDROME
Intrauterine rubella infections often produce severe malformation of the fetus, leading to mental deficiency, cardiovascular disorders, deafness, and other disorders. The most dramatic ophthalmoscopic finding is the pigmentary variation referred to as salt-and-pepper retinopathy that is characterized by widespread fundus changes that simulate congenital syphilis, blunt trauma, and retinitis pigmentosa (Figure 95). Other ocular abnormalities stemming from this infection include microphthalmia, iritis, abnormalities of the pupil, cataracts, and glaucoma.

Miscellaneous
Retinal Disorders

RETROLENTAL FIBROPLASIA

Retrolental fibroplasia is a disease of premature infants exposed to supplementary oxygen. Rarely, it occurs in premature infants who have not been exposed to supplementary oxygen, and very rarely is it reported in full-term infants. The retinal blood vessels are known to be extremely sensitive to high oxygen concentrations; they react with marked vasoconstriction. In the adult, this reaction is reversible, and the vessels will dilate when the oxygen level returns to normal. However, when the immature retinal blood vessel is exposed to prolonged high oxygen levels, there is permanent constriction and eventual occlusion of the vessel. It is not known if this destructive process is secondary to the direct effects of the oxygen or to ischemia produced by the marked and prolonged vasoconstriction. Subsequently, there is a vasoproliferative response with an associated glial reaction. This leads to scarring and traction on the retina. At the time of birth, the temporal retinal blood vessels are very immature and hence are most sensitive to oxygen exposure. Therefore, subsequent vasoproliferation and traction will drag the macula temporally, and this can be seen ophthalmoscopically (Figure 96). Although many cases of retrolental fibroplasia are minimal and asymptomatic, the more severe cases can produce a marked decrease in vision by the dragging and distortion of the macular photoreceptors. Many asymptomatic cases are detected by careful retinal examination and confirmed by a history of prematurity and supplementary oxygen exposure. Blindness may result from irreparable retinal detachments. Retrolental fibroplasia may be prevented by controlling the amount of supplementary oxygen administered and by monitoring the infant's arterial oxygen level.

COATS' DISEASE

Coats' disease is an exudative retinopathy of unknown origin associated with vascular changes (Figures 64 and 97). Coats' disease displays massive subretinal (lipid) exudation secondary to telangiectatic vascular abnormalities. Microaneurysms and aneurysmal dilatation of vascular walls are predominant findings, but there are also areas of capillary avascularity. These vascular changes tend to occur temporally, especially in the superior quadrant.

Coats' disease usually occurs in young males and tends to be monocular. The fluorescein and angiographic changes are dramatic, demonstrating the aneurysms, capillary dilatations, avascular areas, and A/V collateral channels. Patients with Coats' disease may be treated by photocoagulation, cryotherapy, and sometimes by a scleral buckling procedure when detachment occurs.

EALES' DISEASE

Eales' disease was first described toward the end of the

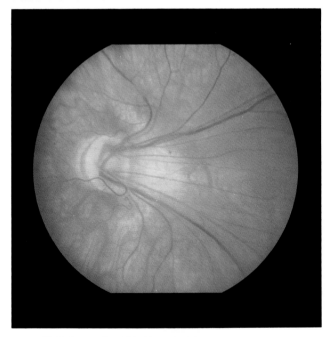

Figure 96. Right eye of a child with *retrolental fibroplasia*. Notice the temporal traction of the retina signaled by the abnormal course of the vasculature extending from the nerve head.

Figure 97A. Illustration of Coats' disease, an acquired progressive abnormality of the vasculature (arrow), accompanied by large amounts of hard intraretinal exudate and often hemorrhage.

Figure 97C. Another patient showing a similar vascular anomaly that has been treated with light coagulation.

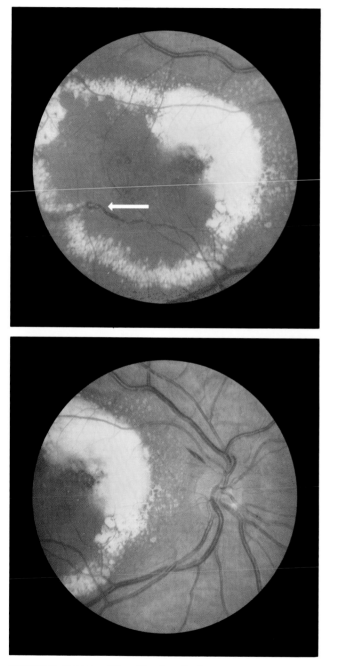

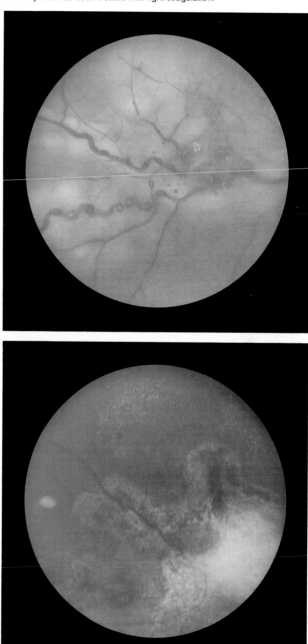

Figure 97B. Same eye, different location, showing Coats' disease.

Figure 97D. The same general area of the fundus as Figure 97C after scarring and vascular obliteration of lesions that would have led to vitreous hemorrhage.

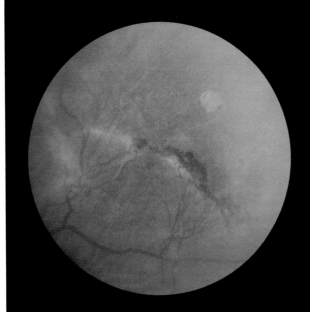

98A.

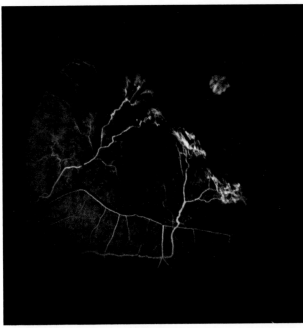

98B.

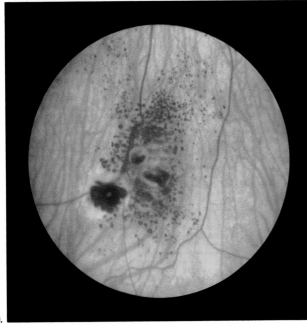

99.

Figure 98A. *Eales' disease* in an otherwise healthy person with progressive retinal ischemic process (usually in the peripheral retina) associated with recurrent vitreous hemorrhage and neovascular proliferation.

Figure 98B. Same fundus as Figure 98A. This illustration is one from a rapid sequence of photographs of a fluorescein angiogram.

Figure 99. Isolated vascular anomalies of the fundus include the occasional cavernous hemangioma associated with multiple tiny aneurysms seen in the peripheral retina.

Figure 100A. A hemangioma of the choroid is seen as an elevated lesion. The vascular nature is demonstrated by the following illustration, Figure 100B.

Figure 100B. Fluorescein angiogram demonstrates the vascular nature of this lesion. Color film has been used for the angiogram.

Figure 101A. Another patient displays a cavernous hemangioma at the margin of the nerve head.

Figure 101B. This patient has a large hemangioma of the optic nerve head itself.

Figure 102A. A fundus area of diabetic retinopathy is illustrated to demonstrate the proliferation of new vessels on the surface of the retina, associated with some hemorrhage.

Figure 102B. The same fundus is shown shortly after multiple bursts of argon laser therapy have been directed to that portion of the retina – in order to occlude the neovascularization and thereby prevent otherwise inevitable hemorrhages and retinal traction.

19th century. Its initial description has not been significantly improved upon, and the etiology of this disorder remains unknown. The disease, basically, is a vasculitis of the retinal veins, beginning in the periphery and extending toward the posterior pole. Ophthalmoscopically, sheathing as well as retinal and preretinal hemorrhages may extend into the vitreous (Figure 98). Such recurrent retinal and vitreous hemorrhages associated with peripheral periphlebitis usually suggest the diagnosis of Eales' disease. Histologic studies show occluded vessels and retinitis proliferans. Eales' disease usually occurs in young males under age 40. Although some of these patients have neurologic deficits, there is no known relationship to a disseminated vasculitis. The literature is replete with reports of a high incidence of positive tuberculin skin testing in patients with Eales' disease; however, there is no evidence of a direct relationship between the two. Photocoagulation has been used to obliterate the neovascular fronds and to diminish the likelihood of recurrent hemorrhages.

OTHER VASCULAR ANOMALIES

Congenital anomalies of the fundus resulting from embryological defects have been mentioned earlier (page 57). Hemangiomas of the retina (Figure 99) are uncommon findings but striking in appearance and are a potential cause of intraocular bleeding. The same is true of hemangiomas of the choroid (Figure 100) and the even rarer hemangiomas of the nerve head (Figure 101). The way that vascular abnormalities of the fundus sometimes are managed is shown in Figure 102.

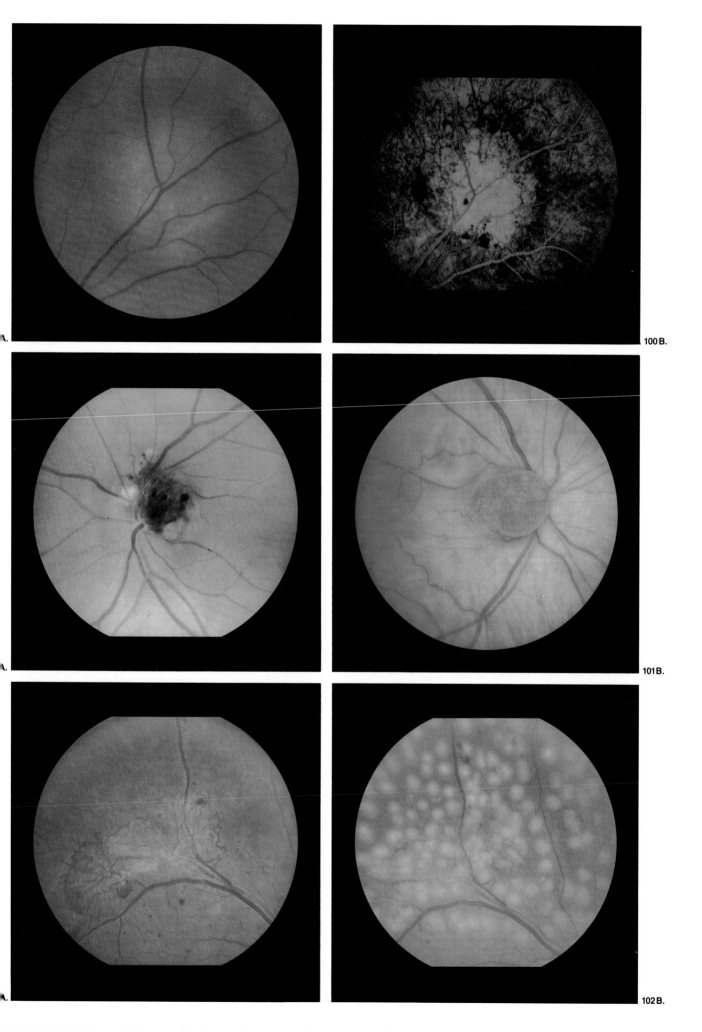

A.

100 B.

A.

101 B.

A.

102 B.

62

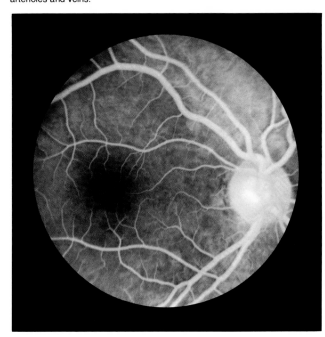

Figure 103. Lipemia retinalis in a diabetic patient with high levels of serum lipid and poor control of his blood sugar. Note the yellow discoloration of the arterioles and veins.

HYPERLIPIDEMIA

Hyperlipidemia occurs in a group of disorders, both familial and acquired, that affect about 20% of the population. The disease is characterized by an increase in concentrations of plasma cholesterol or triglycerides (or both). The lipid constituents of the plasma are cholesterol, triglycerides, and phospholipids. From a clinical point of view, only the cholesterol and triglycerides are considered in the classification of these disorders. The plasma phospholipids do not travel freely and are bound to protein. By means of ultracentrifugation and electrophoresis, the lipoproteins have been divided into four major groups. The blood lipids are derived from the diet, preexistent adipose deposits, and endogenous synthesis. The liver synthesizes most of the alpha- and prebeta-lipoproteins while the chylomicrons are derived from the gut.

The ocular manifestations of hyperlipidemia include corneal arcus, xanthomata (xanthelasmas), and *lipemia retinalis* (Figure 103). Corneal arcus is frequently seen in patients with types IV, V, and especially type II hyperlipoproteinemia. Xanthelasmas are sometimes seen in the type II disorder. The eruptive xanthomata and lipemia retinalis are seen in types I and V when the triglyceride level is elevated above 2,000 mg%.

The ophthalmoscopic appearance of *lipemia retinalis* is dramatic. The entire fundus, including the vessel, acquires a yellow, creamy color. With dietary treatment and medications that lower the serum lipids, a remarkable clearing of the retinal lipemia will occur. Thus, the finding of *lipemia retinalis* is evanescent, and the appearance one day may be markedly different the next.

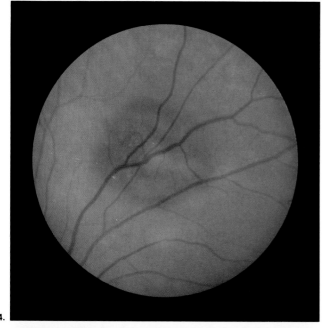

Pigmented Lesions of the Fundus

Pigmented lesions include a multitude of diagnostic fundus entities. We will consider nevi, melanomas, melanocytomas, and pigment epithelial hypertrophy. It is incumbent upon any physician detecting a pigmented lesion of doubtful type to obtain the opinion of an ophthalmologist.

CHOROIDAL NEVI

The synonymous terms *nevus* and *benign melanoma* refer to a lesion composed of dense choroidal melanocytes. These collections of melanocytes only rarely become malignant. Sometimes they increase in pigmentation during puberty or pregnancy. On fundus examination, they are seen as flat, gray, or greenish-gray lesions, often with feathery or indistinct borders (Figure 104). Although these lesions may be slightly elevated, there is no distortion of the overlying retina; consequently, there is no alteration in visual acuity nor is there a visual field defect. Sometimes, drusen are seen on the surface of the nevus, but there is no hemorrhage, surrounding edema, or variation in the degree of pigmentation of its surface. Most nevi are one to three disc diameters in greatest dimension. Should any doubt exist as to the benign nature of the lesion, it is advisable to have fundus photography and fluorescein angiography obtained. Nevi must be differentiated from the more serious malignant melanoma.

Dense *black* spots of comparable size and unrelated to any other fundus pathology are more unusual and constitute benign hypertrophy of the retinal pigment epithelium (Figures 105 and 106). Malignancy need not be suspected in these lesions.

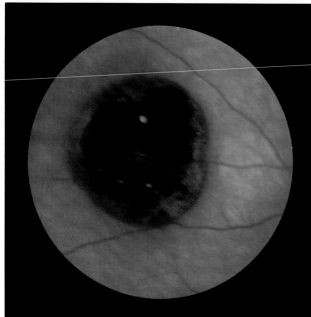

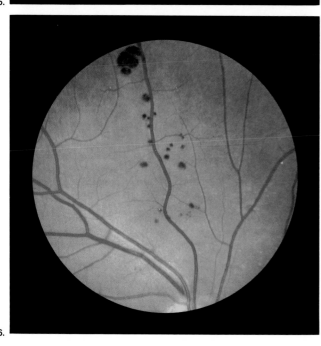

Figure 104. A benign choroidal *nevus.*

Figure 105. The large black lesion is benign *hypertrophy of the retinal pigment epithelium.*

Figure 106. *"Bear track" congenital pigmentation* of the fundus constitutes an incidental finding of no significance.

64

MALIGNANT MELANOMA

Malignant melanomas are derived from the melanocytes or Schwann's cells of the uveal tract and are the most common malignant intraocular tumors. Although these tumors may arise from the iris, ciliary body, or choroid, they occur more frequently in the posterior portions of the choroid. Melanomas do not have a demonstrable genetic predisposition; they are rare in children and in pigmented races and are diagnosed most frequently in patients fifty years of age and older. Ophthalmoscopically, melanomas appear as pigmented masses varying in size and pigmentation, elevating the retina, and protruding into the vitreous (Figures 107, 108, 109, and 110). Some malignant melanomas of the choroid are amelanotic. As these tumors grow, they mushroom through Bruch's membrane (Figure 109) and may produce a detachment of the overlying retina.

Melanomas must be differentiated from subretinal hemorrhages, serous detachments, chorioretinal inflammation, and other intraocular tumors. Intravenously administered radioactive phosphorus, followed by a measurement of radioactivity of the tumor by means of a counterprobe placed on the sclera posterior to the tumor, affords more than 95% accuracy in the diagnosis of a malignant tumor. Recent experimental work indicates that detection of circulating tumor antibodies, as well as a positive skin reaction to a soluble extract of melanoma cells, may serve as diagnostic tests in the future. The patient's prognosis depends on the tissue type of the tumor, determined after enucleation. Patients with ocular melanomas may die of metastatic disease, the liver being the most common site of metastases. Conversely, it is extremely rare for a cutaneous melanoma to metastasize to the eye.

Although the classic surgical treatment of a progressive or large melanoma is enucleation, this should not be done until two or more ophthalmologists concur with the clinical diagnosis. These tumors have been treated conservatively with extraocular radioactive gold plaques or with radon seeds in combination with photocoagulation of the lesion. Some results seem favorable if the tumor is small, but if the other eye is normal, enucleation of the eye affected with certain malignant melanoma remains the usual management.

Recently there is increasing conservatism in the management of melanomas. The lesion should be seven or more disc diameters in size, elevated, and known to be growing before removal of the eye is clearly indicated.

MELANOCYTOMA OF THE OPTIC NERVE HEAD

Melanocytomas are locally invasive, nonmalignant tumors arising at the optic disc from uveal melanocytes. In contradistinction to malignant melanomas, they occur more frequently in non-Caucasians, and usually do not produce visual symptoms or field defects. Ophthalmoscopically, they have a very characteristic appearance: small and evenly pigmented and only rarely bulging into the vitreous. They usually occur in a lower temporal quadrant of the disc (Figure 111). Locally, these tumors may infiltrate to the lamina cribrosa or into the adjacent retina and choroid. It is important to be aware of this invariably benign tumor in order to prevent unnecessary enucleation which might otherwise be performed because of suspected malignant melanoma. Radioactive P_{32} uptake studies are difficult to perform because of the location of the optic nerve head. Ultrasonography may be helpful in assessing the size and determining whether changes occur during the follow-up period, but periodic fundus photography is the most helpful and available means for precise follow-up comparisons. There is no treatment for these tumors, and usually none is required.

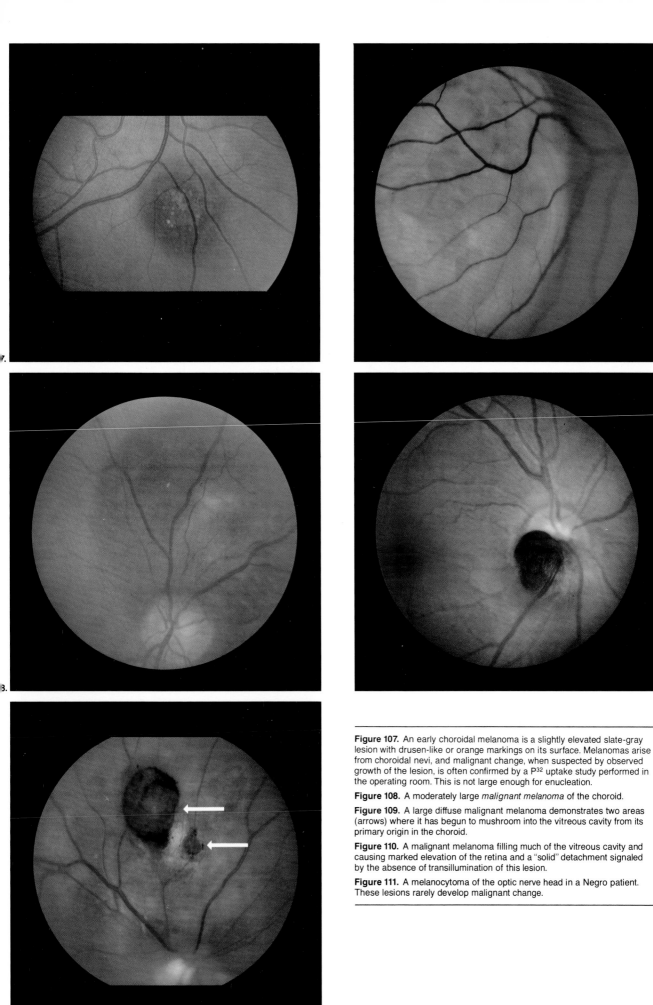

Figure 107. An early choroidal melanoma is a slightly elevated slate-gray lesion with drusen-like or orange markings on its surface. Melanomas arise from choroidal nevi, and malignant change, when suspected by observed growth of the lesion, is often confirmed by a P³² uptake study performed in the operating room. This is not large enough for enucleation.

Figure 108. A moderately large *malignant melanoma* of the choroid.

Figure 109. A large diffuse malignant melanoma demonstrates two areas (arrows) where it has begun to mushroom into the vitreous cavity from its primary origin in the choroid.

Figure 110. A malignant melanoma filling much of the vitreous cavity and causing marked elevation of the retina and a "solid" detachment signaled by the absence of transillumination of this lesion.

Figure 111. A melanocytoma of the optic nerve head in a Negro patient. These lesions rarely develop malignant change.

Retinal Detachments

Retinal detachments constitute a separation of the sensory retina from the underlying retinal pigment epithelium, due to the accumulation of fluid in that potential space. Most retinal detachments are the result of one or more retinal holes that allow passage of fluid between the sensory retina and the pigment epithelium. The detachment may remain quite flat or it may become large and bullous – in which case it protrudes into the vitreous cavity (Figure 112). Detachments may occur anywhere in the retina wherever the hole is located (Figure 113). Superior detachments are more serious than inferior detachments because they may rapidly extend inferiorly to detach the macula with loss of central vision that may be permanent, even if surgery is successful in restoring the retina to its proper position.

Symptoms associated with a retinal detachment may be minimal. Usually the patient complains of light flashes, dark floating specks, and a curtain-like defect in the field of vision. Such complaints should lead to

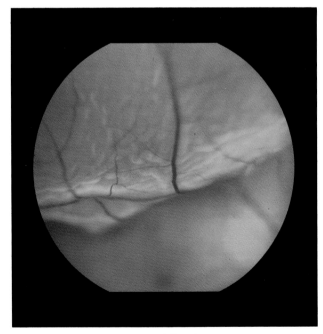

Figure 112. This fundus view shows a billowed *detachment of the retina* with the posterior portion of the fundus out of focus.

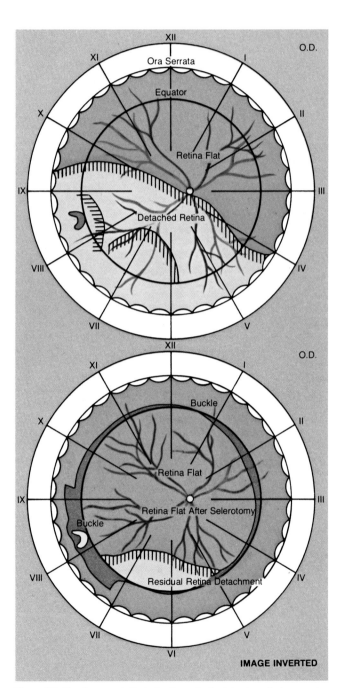

Figure 113. The diagrams indicate the type of retinal drawings that are made by ophthalmologists involved in the surgical repair of retinal detachments. In the upper figure, there is a single retinal tear that has led to a detachment of almost half of the retina (indicated by blue color). In the bottom figure, an encircling buckle has been placed around the eye. The hole has been sealed by this buckle and will form a scar between the retina and choroid as a result of cryo applications. The residual retinal detachment (blue), shown posterior to the buckle, will promptly resorb and the entire retina will again be restored to its proper position.

prompt referral to an ophthalmologist. Light flashes and floaters alone are less ominous and usually signal vitreous detachment from the retina which occurs symptomatically in many adults.

Using the direct ophthalmoscope, a large bullous detachment of the retina is easily recognized. However, many retinal detachments are located principally in the anterior (peripheral) region of the retina which is difficult to observe with the direct ophthalmoscope. This situation requires an examiner who is familiar with the indirect ophthalmoscope, to make the diagnosis; scleral depression is usually necessary. Most retinal detachments are associated with retinal holes (often difficult for the beginner to find), and the holes, in turn, are the result of vitreous traction – best exemplified by the classical horseshoe-shaped tear (Figures 114 and 115).

retina that predispose to hole formation. Highly myopic individuals are more prone to retinal holes and detachments. Following severe trauma to the eye, one may develop a traumatic detachment from vitreous traction resulting from hemorrhage and fibrosis. So-called idiopathic lattice degeneration of the retina often predisposes to retinal holes and subsequent detachments (Figure 116). All of the above detachments, being secondary to a retinal hole or tear, are referred to as *rhegmatogenous detachments*. Rhegma, in Greek, means a hole.

Detachments not secondary to a retinal hole are called *nonrhegmatogenous detachments* and are caused by primary choroidal tumors, inflammation, or metastatic lesions. The tumors that commonly produce these "secondary" detachments are choroidal melanomas or metastatic carcinomas of the breast and lung that migrate to the choroid.

Retinal detachments are repaired by sealing the hole or holes with cryotherapy, diathermy, or photocoagulation. The subretinal fluid may or may not have to be

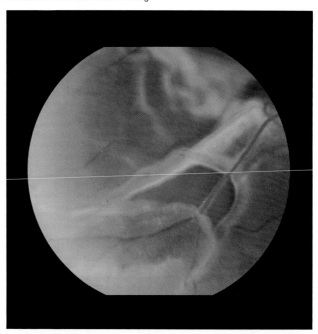

Figure 114. A large horseshoe-shaped retinal tear in the region of the retinal vessel. This illustration indicates why the occurrence of a retinal tear is often associated with intraocular bleeding.

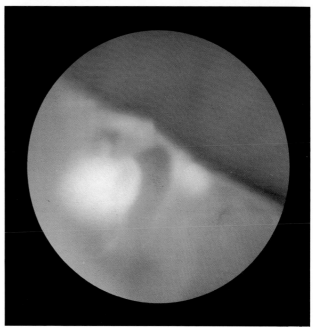

Figure 115. A horseshoe tear in apposition with invaginated choroid and sclera (surgically created "buckle" formed by an encircling element). This illustration corresponds to the treated horseshoe tear shown in the lower left portion of the bottom diagram of Figure 113.

Figure 116A. *Lattice degeneration* of the peripheral retina is a common site for retinal hole formation and may be the origin of a retinal detachment.

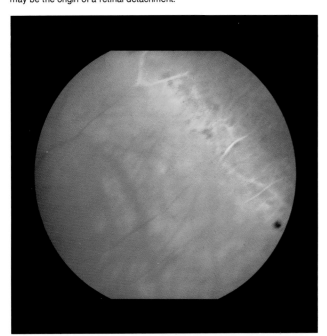

drained, and sometimes a silicone buckle is placed like a belt around the globe to facilitate closure of the hole (Figure 113). Ninety-five percent of rhegmatogenous detachments can be cured by prompt surgical intervention. Detachments secondary to underlying tumors have to be managed by considering treatment of the tumor itself: enucleation with primary tumors (not known to have metastasized), and occasionally helpful radiation, and/or chemotherapy with secondary tumors.

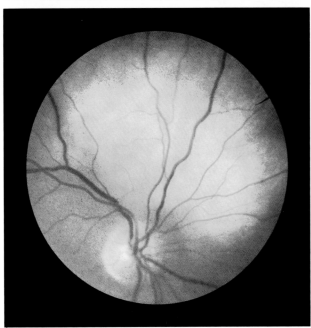

Figure 116B. Retinal detachment may occur without a retinal hole when due to a metastatic tumor (as above), or to inflammation of the choroid.

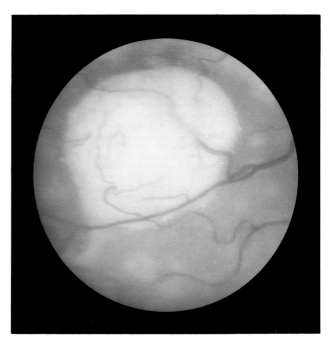

Figure 117. *Retinoblastomas* can have single or multiple origins within the same eye.

Retinoblastoma

Retinoblastoma is the most common intraocular tumor of childhood. Current statistics show that it occurs annually in ten children per million under the age of five. This tumor may be classified as familial or sporadic. Survivors of retinoblastoma who bear children show an autosomal dominant mode of tumor transmission with incomplete penetrance. Sporadic retinoblastomas characterize 94% to 96% of cases.

Retinoblastomas arise from undifferentiated retinal epithelial cells or from glial cells; both eyes are affected in about 50% of cases. These tumors frequently originate from the inner layer of the retina although multiple sites of tumor development are not unusual. The tumor may spread in the eye via the vitreous or subretinal fluid.

Ophthalmoscopically, retinoblastomas are elevated white masses (Figure 117) that may show radiopaque deposits of calcium (Figure 118). Growing rapidly, they may fill much of the vitreous cavity, making the pupil appear white (*leukocoria*). In the differential diagnosis of leukocoria, one must consider congenital cataract, retinal detachment, congenital retinal folds, nematode infections, persistence of primary vitreous, retrolental fibroplasia, and other abnormalities. A child with a retinoblastoma may present with a white pupil, recent onset of strabismus, unilateral glaucoma, uveitis, or iris neovascularization with secondary hyphema.

Recently, it has been shown that an elevated lactic acid dehydrogenase content of the aqueous is highly suggestive of retinoblastoma, and this may prove useful in diagnosis.

Favorable prognostic signs include solitary small tumors located posterior to the equator. Multiple large tumors extending anterior to the ora serrata with vitreous seeding carry a poor prognosis. The usual form of treatment for monocular cases is enucleation; the survival rate is related to whether there has been extraocular extension prior to enucleation. Orbital involvement

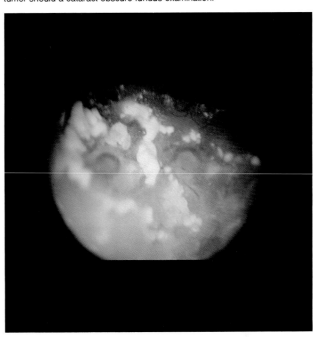

Figure 118. Calcium deposition in a retinoblastoma is demonstrated and explains the presence of radio-opacities, sometimes helpful in the diagnosis of this tumor should a cataract obscure fundus examination.

is managed by exenteration of all orbital tissues. Other modes of treatment include irradiation and chemotherapy. Successful treatment of small tumors by photocoagulation has been reported. Death usually occurs secondary to direct extension to the central nervous system via the optic nerve as well as by metastatic complications. Fortunately, most cases recognized early and treated appropriately are no longer fatal.

Intraocular Foreign Bodies

The most common retained intraocular foreign body is a chip of metal that often is the result of a hammering accident. The small metallic foreign body usually penetrates through the anterior segment of the eye and may be found in the vitreous (Figure 119), or may lodge on the retina (Figure 120). It is important that surgical removal be accomplished promptly; long-term retention of steel-containing metallic chips will lead to siderosis; copper-containing foreign bodies will lead to chalcosis. In some instances, the foreign body enters the eye with little or no associated bleeding, and visualization with the direct ophthalmoscope is readily accomplished, as indicated in the two illustrations. Should hemorrhage obscure visualization, accurate localization can be accomplished by special radiological techniques or ultrasonography. Magnetic foreign bodies are usually removed readily by the use of a giant magnet; nonmagnetic foreign bodies must be removed by grasping them with foreign body forceps, using direct visualization at the time of surgery.

Figure 119. A metallic intraocular foreign body on the surface of the retina causing retinal edema in the area of its impact (arrow).

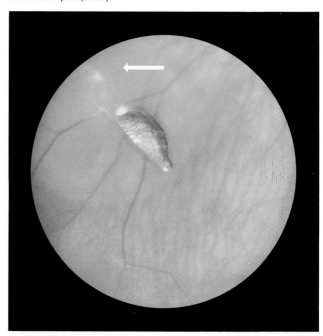

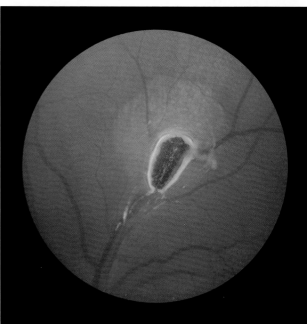

Figure 120. Metallic foreign body lodged within the retina with a halo of surrounding edema.

Acquired Macular Disorders

The following macular abnormalities are acquired or are nonhereditary degenerative disorders.

RETINAL PIGMENT EPITHELIAL DETACHMENTS
The retinal pigment epithelium is firmly attached to Bruch's membrane of the choroid. A lesion or degenerative change of that membrane sometimes leads to a local elevation or detachment of the pigment epithelium. A defect in Bruch's membrane may allow a serous or hemorrhagic exudation from the choroid to detach the pigment epithelium. These detachments are usually unilateral and solitary. However, in some patients there may be multiple retinal pigment epithelial detachments involving both eyes. Ophthalmoscopically, these detachments appear to be discrete, local elevations (Figures 121 and 122). If the detachments are long-standing, an overlying pigmentary alteration may develop, which aids in its recognition. These detachments are of no significance unless they involve the macular area or lead to a larger serous detachment between the pigment epithelium and the layer of rods and cones.

A retinal pigment epithelial detachment away from the macular area produces no visual symptoms. With proximity to the macula, it may interfere with visual acuity or produce a scotoma and visual field defect. Patients sometimes complain of *metamorphopsia*, a symptom in which straight lines or figures appear distorted. If a retinal pigment epithelial detachment is not symptomatic, it should be observed and followed, not treated. If the detachment encroaches upon the macular area, it may be treated by photocoagulation, taking care not to damage the fovea.

CENTRAL SEROUS CHOROIDOPATHY
Central serous choroidopathy is basically a choroidal disease of unknown etiology; it has been referred to in the older literature as central angiospastic retinopathy. It is thought that some alteration in the choroidal cir-

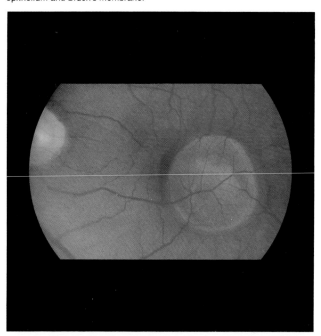

Figure 121. The smooth-walled elevated and translucent lesion encroaching upon the macula is a detachment of the retinal pigment epithelium. Serous fluid has accumulated between the pigment epithelium and Bruch's membrane.

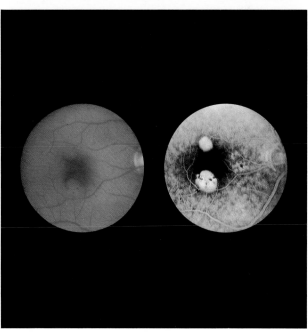

Figure 122. Another retinal pigment epithelium detachment is shown, left, along with the fluorescein angiogram, right, demonstrating diffuse fluorescence of the small detachments.

culation or change in retinal pigment epithelial permeability allows a serous exudate to detach the retina (between the epithelium and the layer of rods and cones). It has been postulated that the etiology of the vascular or permeability defect is allergic or autoimmune, but these theories remain unproven. These are called *serous detachments* and are more common in males (age 30 to 50) undergoing excessive emotional stress at the time of their symptoms. The initial symptom usually is a wavy distortion of the central vision, metamorphopsia, and a noticeable blind spot or scotoma. There may be a mild or moderate drop in the visual acuity.

The ophthalmoscopic picture is characterized by a visible but subtle detachment of the retina in the macular area – well circumscribed and slightly elevated – with a decrease in the superficial retinal reflex (Figure 123). Occasionally, one can detect an accompanying detachment of the pigment epithelium. The prognosis for recovery of these detachments is quite good and many of them regress spontaneously. Most ophthalmologists observe these detachments for a period of months before initiating any therapy other than mild sedation or tranquilizers. Medical treatment with corticosteroids seems to be of little value. If the visual acuity remains diminished for months, laser treatment may be indicated, particularly if the leakage site is extrafoveal. Successful photocoagulation is dependent upon identifying and sealing the leakage sites. Fluorescein angiography is indispensable in distinguishing these leaks from the choroid that account for the accumulation of serous fluid between sensory retina and pigment epithelium. The fluorescein angiogram is characteristic and localized, showing at least one small pinhead leak that slowly grows in size as the fluorescein diffuses throughout the detachment (Figure 123B). An early phase of leakage is demonstrated here; as seen in Figure 123A, the detachment itself occupies most of the posterior pole.

Figure 123A. Central serous choroidopathy is demonstrated in this illustration showing the clinical appearance of the lesion.

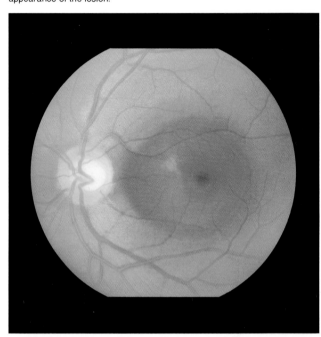

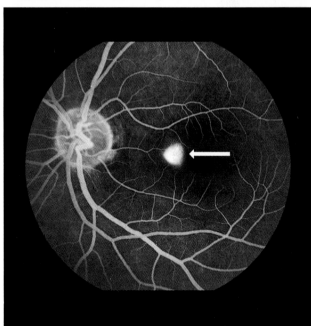

Figure 123B. In the fluorescein angiogram, serous fluid from the choroid has broken through the retinal pigment epithelium, and leakage of dye into the macular detachment is shown in an early phase of dissemination (arrow).

Figure 124A. Early senile macular degeneration with a predominance of drusen and no hemorrhages, left eye.

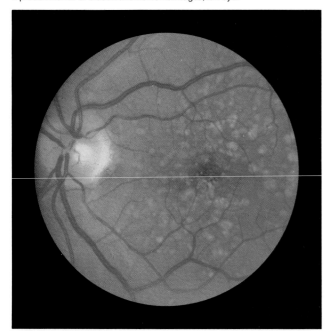

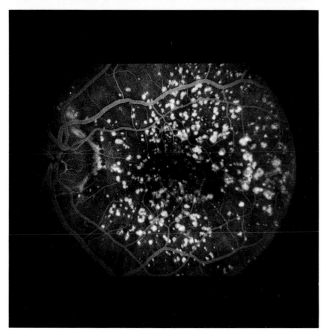

Figure 124B. Angiogram of Figure 124A.

SENILE MACULAR DEGENERATION

For the patient's sake, a physician shows more empathy if he uses the slightly more sophisticated word "senescent" than "senile" when describing either the cataracts or this form of macular degeneration. Regardless, senile macular degeneration is the common verbage, and it constitutes the leading cause of "blindness" in the United States. (Note that blindness is defined as a visual acuity of 20/200 or less, and this means that a patient may have normal peripheral vision and be legally blind.)

Senile macular degeneration is preceded by age-related changes in the posterior fundus. In most cases, there is both a mottling of the retinal pigment epithelium at the posterior pole and scattered drusen (Figure 124). Degenerative changes at the level of Bruch's membrane lead to thickening of that membrane, colloid excrescences (drusen), and eventually to leakage of fluid and blood into the retina from the choroid's capillary layer (choriocapillaris). Small serous detachments of the retinal pigment epithelium occur, and these are often followed by neovascular membranes extending from the choriocapillaris to the space between Bruch's membrane and the pigment epithelium (Figure 125). These vessels cause transudation, hemorrhage, a fibrous tissue proliferation, and destruction of the sensory retina at the posterior pole. The end stage of this process is the occurrence of an elevated macular scar, disciform macular degeneration (Figure 126).

In the past, vasodilators and multivitamins have been recommended as treatment for senile macular degeneration, although these forms of therapy have been of no demonstrable value. In recent years, the use of photocoagulation, especially with the laser, has been directed at treating the neovascular membranes and leakage sites. The long-range benefits are not impressive in the majority of cases.

74

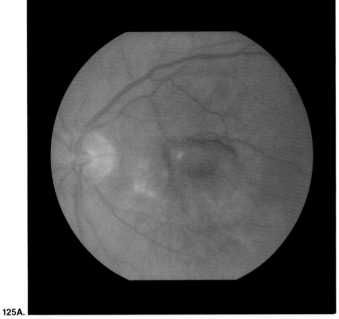

125A.

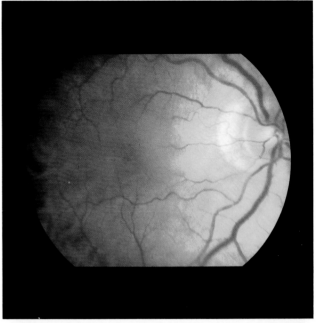

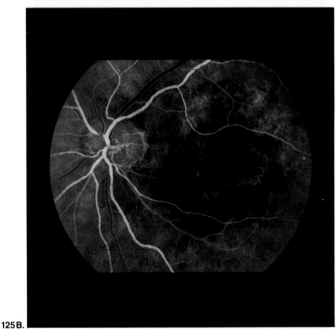

125B.

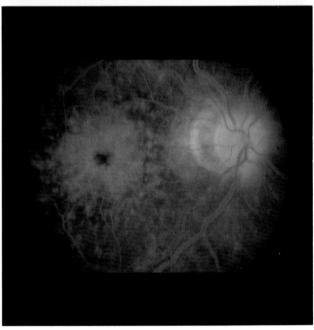

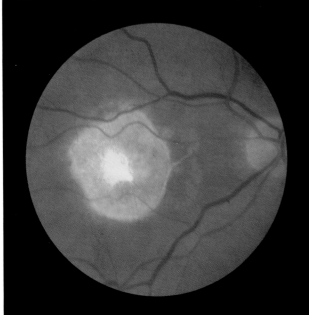

126.

Figure 125A. *Senile macular degeneration* is often accompanied by macular hemorrhage resulting from the growth of new vessels extending from the choroid into the retina. Extensive hemorrhagic degeneration and scar tissue proliferation often ensue.

Figure 125B. Fluorescein angiography demonstrates neovascularization.

Figure 126. A so-called *disciform degeneration of the macula* constitutes the end stage of senile macular degeneration. The same macular scar is seen in patients with long-standing angioid streaks.

Figure 127A. The macula of patients with *Irvine-Gass syndrome* shows a loss of foveal reflex and vague impression of macular edema.

Figure 127B. The fluorescein angiogram in the same patient demonstrates intraretinal edema in a pattern pathognomonic of the Irvine-Gass syndrome.

CHOROIDAL NEOVASCULAR MEMBRANES

A choroidal neovascular membrane is a tuft of choroidal capillaries and connective tissue extending from the choroid through Bruch's membrane. These neovascular tufts insinuate between Bruch's membrane and the pigment epithelium or actually under the sensory retina. Ophthalmoscopically, suspicion of their presence is raised by the observation of a dirty gray or yellow elevated patch beneath the retina (Figure 125). The diagnosis of a choroidal neovascular membrane is confirmed by fluorescein angiography, with the neovascular membrane appearing as an irregular spoked-wheel lesion in the subretinal space. Choroidal neovascular membranes may be seen in the macular area associated with senile macular degeneration, angioid streaks, myopic degeneration, choroidal tumors, and the ocular histoplasmosis syndrome. Neovascular membranes may produce a severe loss of vision through hemorrhages and/or by producing a serous detachment. Presently, the only form of treatment is photocoagulation to obliterate the membrane and, hence, diminish the likelihood of a hemorrhagic or serous detachment, but only if the treatment can be accomplished without destruction of the macula.

CYSTOID MACULOPATHY

If one looks carefully, *cystoid maculopathy* will be found in approximately 30% of patients who have had recent cataract surgery. Moreover, peripheral retinal and vitreous inflammation (an entity referred to as *pars planitis* or *chronic peripheral retinitis*) has a rather high incidence of cystoid maculopathy in the lengthy course of this disease of unknown etiology. When occurring following cataract extraction, this transient phenomenon is referred to as the *Irvine-Gass syndrome*. The patient complains of minimal or moderate loss of central visual acuity unassociated with other symptoms. The presenting request is that the ophthalmolo-

gist provide a change of glasses. Fundus examination reveals multilobulated, fine cystoid changes that affect the macula and are sometimes associated with surrounding retinal edema (Figure 127). Although in the majority of cases the diagnosis is usually made by ophthalmoscopic examination, the fluorescein angiogram is pathognomonic and extremely helpful when fundus examination is difficult or the lesion is very early. Not only is there leakage of fluorescein into the retina but also leakage of dye from the optic nerve head is often observed. In some patients with this disease entity, treatment with systemic corticosteroids seems effective whereas in others no medication has demonstrable effect. The majority of retinas with mild cystoid maculopathy have spontaneous regression and restoration of normal acuity.

TRAUMATIC MACULAR SCARS, RUPTURES, HOLES, AND EDEMA

Direct trauma to the eye may produce hemorrhage (Figure 128) that may resorb completely or may be followed by a pigmentary alteration at the macula with variable degrees of visible scar tissue (Figure 129). Histologically, the scar is composed of glial reaction, atrophic retinal and pigmentary elements. These scars may have a severe effect on the visual acuity, but often, after the hemorrhage has cleared, the majority of the central vision is still retained.

Accompanying the retinal scar may be a rupture of the underlying choroid, including Bruch's membrane. Trauma-induced choroidal ruptures occur concentric with the optic nerve head, or traverse beneath the macula in a generally vertical direction. Ophthalmoscopically, choroidal ruptures appear as yellowish, homogenous, curvilinear lines, and are relatively easy to diagnose once the initial hemorrhage has cleared (Figure 130). Occasionally, a choroidal rupture will lead to a vascular tuft proliferating through the rupture. Such

Figure 128. A trauma-induced hemorrhage has occurred under the pigment epithelium at the posterior pole, with dissection of blood into more superficial retinal layers at the periphery of the hemorrhage.

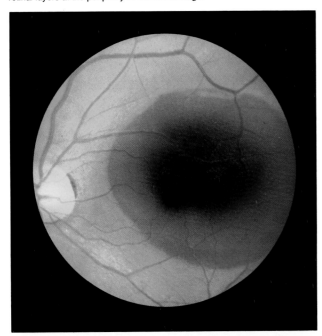

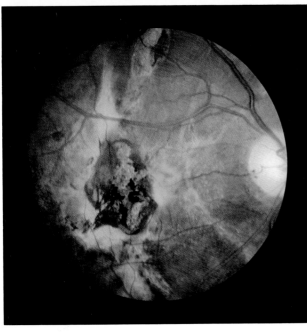

Figure 129. Severe blunt trauma to the eye often causes extensive hemorrhages. As these resolve, *choroidal ruptures* (the origin of the deep hemorrhages) appear as curvilinear yellow-white scars.

neovascular choroidal membranes (page 75) may subsequently hemorrhage and elevate the retina. Sometimes the choroidal response is more fibrotic than vascular, forming a subretinal glial membrane. Although a choroidal rupture is not amenable to treatment, associated choroidal neovascular membranes may be obliterated by photocoagulation.

Macular holes are usually caused by trauma or long-standing macular edema but may be idiopathic (presumably from vitreous traction). Histologic studies of macular holes have revealed that they are either partial or full thickness. Ophthalmoscopically, it is quite difficult to differentiate between a partial or full-thickness macular hole. However, with the aid of a slit lamp and an examining contact lens, differentiation is less difficult. Fluorescein angiography may demonstrate the presence of a hole, but it will not differentiate a partial from a full thickness hole. From a visual point of view, whether the hole is partial or full thickness is unimportant. In either situation, there is usually a loss of central vision and an accompanying central scotoma. The degree of visual acuity and visual field loss is commensurate with the size of the hole. Therapeutically, there is no restorative treatment. Usually, these macular holes are not associated with a retinal detachment (Figure 131).

Occasionally, after direct ocular contusion, retinal edema may develop at the posterior pole or in the periphery. Ophthalmoscopically, a diffuse white edematous retina is visible (Figure 132). Visual acuity slowly improves as the retinal edema declines. A history of recent trauma usually helps to confirm the diagnosis of contusion injury.

A more severe concussion injury caused by the nearby passage of a bullet can cause extensive damage to the choroid and retina and is termed *retinitis sclopeteria* (Figure 133). Severe traumatic displacement of the globe causes a different type of serious traumatic injury, avulsion of the nerve (Figure 134).

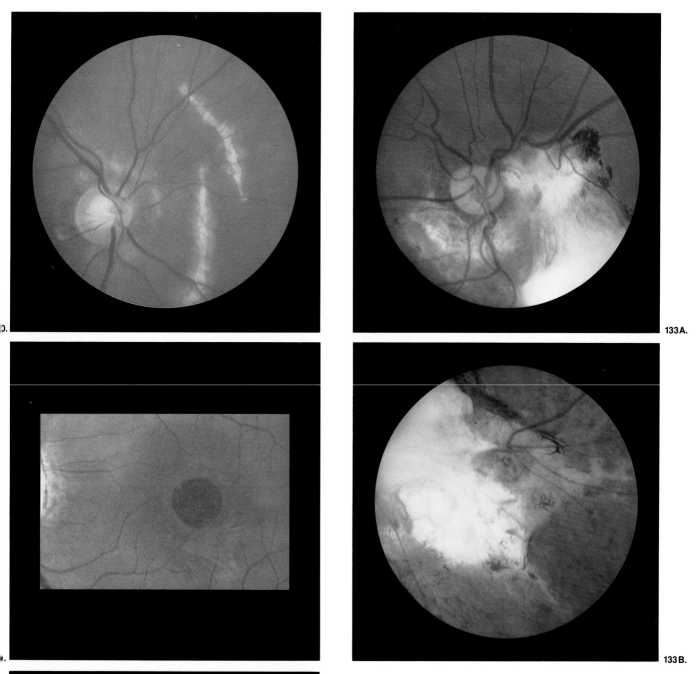

133A.

133B.

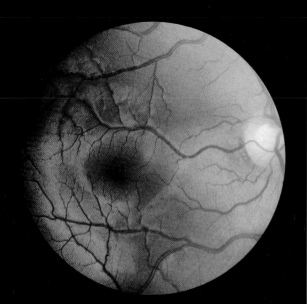

Figure 130. In Figure 129, choroidal ruptures extend through the macula with associated fibrovascular scarring. In this illustration of choroidal ruptures, nasal to the optic nerve head, only the scarring of the rupture is seen.

Figure 131. A *macular hole* may be "idiopathic," or may follow edema, inflammation, or trauma. The slit beam of the direct ophthalmoscope is helpful in demonstrating the concavity of the hole.

Figure 132. Diffuse or localized edema of the retina can occur from blunt trauma alone, as shown in this patient demonstrating *commotio retinae*.

Figure 133A. Retinitis sclopteria is a form of traumatic chorioretinopathy caused in this case by the nearby passage of a bullet as a result of a hunting accident. It is a form of concussion injury to the eye resulting in severe damage to retinal function.

Figure 133B. Figures 133A and 133B are the same fundus at different locations. Vision is 5/200.

Figure 134. Sudden distortion of the globe has led to an avulsion of the optic nerve head, shown after hemorrhage has resorbed.

Figure 136. The long-term use of chloroquine can lead to a toxic retinopathy. The typical *"bull's eye"* appearance of the macula is illustrated.

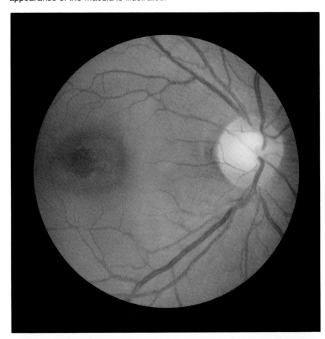

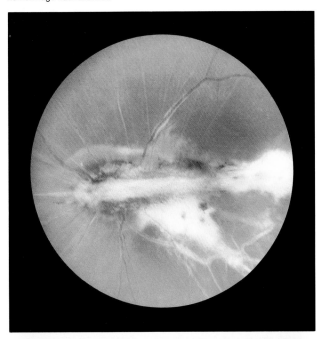

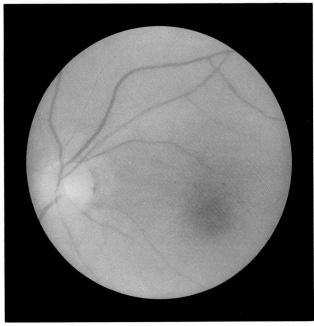

Figure 135. Solar maculopathy is the result of eclipse watching or sungazing. A subtle change can be seen in this high-power view of the macula.

Figure 137. Other irreversible changes of chloroquine toxicity include narrowing and attenuation of the retinal arterioles and a waxy appearance of the disc.

SOLAR RETINOPATHY

Solar or eclipse retinopathy is an actinic burn of the fovea secondary to either unintentional or intentional sun gazing. This lesion may occur in the casual sun bather, but more characteristically in a person viewing a solar eclipse without proper precaution. Initially, the fovea has a yellow appearance secondary to an exudative response (Figure 135), and often there is perifoveal edema around the fovea. Subsequently, pigmentary alterations develop and frequently a foveal cyst forms. Associated with this ophthalmoscopic appearance is a decrease in visual acuity and a scotoma. During the early stages of the lesion, administration of corticosteroids may reduce the edema and the inflammatory response. A careful history is essential to confirm the diagnosis that is suggested by the foveal appearance.

CHLOROQUINE RETINOPATHY

It is now known that long-term administration of chloroquine may produce pigmentary disturbances at the macula (Figure 136), attenuation of the arterioles, and a waxy appearance of the optic nerve head (Figure 137). This type of retinopathy is not reversible and is the result of a toxic retinal interaction with chloroquine that is directly related to duration and dosage of therapy.

Ophthalmoscopically, the examiner sees a ring-like, depigmented lesion encircling the macula; surrounding this zone of hypopigmentation is a ring of relative hyperpigmentation, hence the term *"bull's eye" maculopathy* as the characteristic but not invariable appearance of the macular disorder. Fluorescein angiography presents a hyperfluorescent appearance through the hypopigmented ring, but there is no active fluorescein leakage. This entity can produce a permanent reduction of central visual acuity as well as extensive paracentral visual field defects.

Patients treated with chloroquine should be seen periodically by an ophthalmologist and cautioned to report immediately any alteration in visual acuity or loss of color sensitivity. The corneal epithelium may have transient chloroquine deposition, causing a halo vision, but it is of no lasting consequence in distinction to the retinal damage. The electroretinogram may be used to detect electrophysiologic abnormalities in the earliest stages of the retinopathy.

80

Hereditary Dystrophies of the Posterior Pole

These dystrophies are heritable conditions that lead to an early retinal cell death. As a group, they have certain common characteristics. The hereditary dystrophies tend to be familial and bilaterally symmetrical and they involve primarily the posterior portion of the fundus. They usually occur at an early age and are characterized by a significant decrease in the visual acuity. The following dystrophies illustrate a variety of retinal appearances.

STARGARDT'S DYSTROPHY
Stargardt's dystrophy primarily involves the retinal neuroepithelium. Affected persons usually have a history of normal vision until the adolescent years at which time they have a gradual decrease in their acuity. Recognizable ophthalmoscopic changes at the onset of visual loss are minimal; subsequently, there is disappearance of the foveal reflex and the development of brownish foveal spots. Eventually, an elliptical area of atrophic pigment epithelium develops that resembles a beaten metal appearance (Figure 138). Concurrently, in some patients, a ring of white spots develops near the macula and may resemble the ophthalmoscopic picture of fundus flavimaculatus.

FUNDUS FLAVIMACULATUS
This posterior pole dystrophy primarily involves the pigment epithelium. It is initially usually detected in young people. The characteristic ophthalmoscopic picture constitutes scattered yellow spots, often shaped like fishtails, from which comes the descriptive term *pisciform* lesions (Figure 139). Over half of these cases show a metallic or beaten bronze appearance at the macula. Thus, the macular change resembles Stargardt's dystrophy.

In Stargardt's dystrophy, the macular involvement is the initial finding, sometimes followed by the development of perimacular spots. By contrast, in fundus

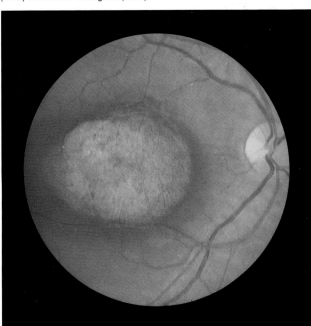

Figure 138. *Stargardt's hereditary macular degeneration* is illustrated by the typical appearance of depigmentation in the posterior pole, obliterating the macula and its function. Compare the similarities with Figure 136. Electrophysiological tests would assist in the differential diagnosis: the electroretinogram (ERG) and electro-oculogram (EOG).

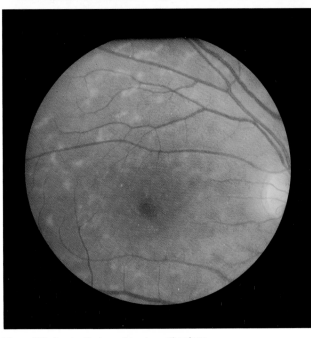

Figure 139. Fundus flavimaculatus is another form of tapetoretinal degeneration affecting the entire retina and easily recognized by the appearance of fishtailed, (pisciform) yellowish lesions scattered throughout the posterior portions of the retina.

flavimaculatus, scattered whitish spots are present before the macular involvement. The visual acuity remains intact if the fovea is not involved. The electro-oculogram (EOG) is characteristically normal. Fluorescein angiography shows multiple retinal pigment epithelial defects.

VITELLIFORM DYSTROPHY

Vitelliform dystrophy of the fovea has been known by many names and eponymically as *Best's disease*. Vitelliform macular changes may or may not be present at birth. Many patients whose fundi appear normal during infancy subsequently develop the macular lesions. Vitelliform dystrophy is usually bilateral, although rare unilateral lesions and asymmetry have been described. Ophthalmoscopically, the vitelliform structure appears to be a yolk-like, round, slightly elevated structure surrounded by a dark border (Figure 140). Usually, the vitelliform lesions evolve into a scrambled egg appearance of retinal scarring (Figure 141) and, although not always present, hyperopia is common. The electroretinogram is usually normal; however, the electro-oculogram, which reflects the function of the retinal pigment epithelium, is distinctly abnormal.

DOMINANT DRUSEN OF BRUCH'S MEMBRANE

In contrast to degenerative drusen (page 22), dominantly inherited drusen of Bruch's membrane are hereditary rather than senescent changes. Histologically, they are eosinophilic, laminated bodies composed of a hyaline material. *Doyne's honeycomb dystrophy* is probably the most common eponym for these inherited drusen. This bilateral condition occurs more frequently in women, and usually the drusen become visible ophthalmoscopically in patients over age 25. The fundus picture is typified by a honeycomb pattern of yellowish-white dots of various sizes at the posterior pole (Figure 142). Eventually, the drusen become confluent. Initially,

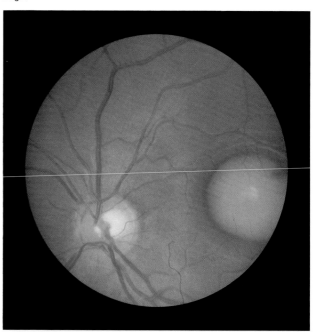

Figure 140. *Vitelliform degeneration of the macula* provides a unique egg-yolk appearance in the early stages.

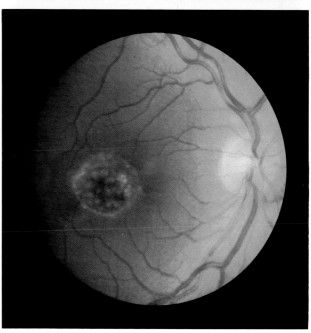

Figure 141. In a later stage of vitelliform degeneration, a "scrambled egg" appearance occurs, but vision may be almost normal.

82

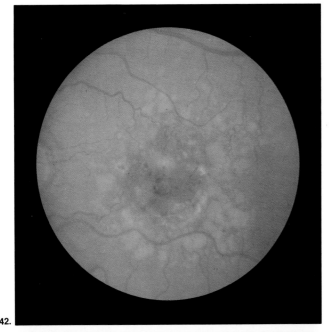

142.

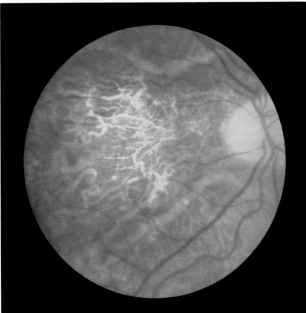

143.

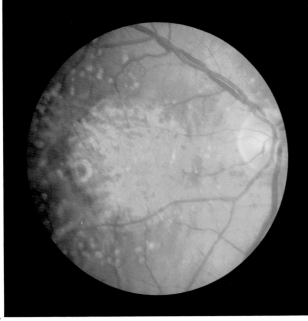

144.

the visual acuity is normal; however, with subsequent retinal and choroidal degeneration, the patient may lose central vision. Although the electroretinograms remain normal, the electro-oculogram ultimately becomes abnormal. Fluorescein angiography shows hyperfluorescence through the "window" defects of pigment epithelium over the drusen, although there is no active leakage of fluorescein.

CENTRAL AREOLAR CHOROIDAL DYSTROPHY
This familial condition, frequently referred to as choroidal sclerosis, is usually detected in young adults. Although initially the visual acuity may be normal, there is often a gradual progression of visual loss, leading to a large central scotoma. The initial lesions are not specific; after a period of time, the pigment epithelium and the choriocapillaris atrophy to such a great extent that the outer large choroidal vessels become plainly visible (Figures 143 and 144). The etiology of this condition is thought to be a dystrophic process of the choroidal vessels.

Figure 142. Drusenoid dystrophy of the macula, similar to Figure 124.

Figure 143. Central areolar choroidal sclerosis is diagnosed by the well-circumscribed atrophy of the retinal pigment epithelium and increased visibility of the choroidal vessels that acquire a white sheathing. Atrophy of the choriocapillaris in this region results in a localized loss of retinal function leading to severe visual impairment.

Figure 144. A similar but more advanced stage of choroidal sclerosis.

Tapetoretinal Degenerations

This group of retinal and choroidal degenerations includes retinitis pigmentosa, choroideremia, and gyrate atrophy. Although their etiology is presently unknown, they have a common bond: all of them produce contraction of the visual fields and night blindness.

RETINITIS PIGMENTOSA

Retinitis pigmentosa is a group of similar disorders with multiple modes of genetic inheritance. The ophthalmoscopic picture is classic (Figures 145 and 146). The earliest ophthalmoscopic signs are jet-black pigment dots, or "bone spicules," located in the equatorial region. These pigmentary changes tend to increase, spreading towards both the periphery and the macula. Usually, the degree of pigmentation is proportionate to the severity of the disease and the visual loss. However, some patients may have severe visual loss with minimal pigmentary changes. Sometimes the pigmentation tends to collect along vessels. Another important ophthalmoscopic finding is progressive attenuation of the retinal vessels, especially of the arterioles. The vessel attenuation is smooth and diffuse with very little caliber variation. The disc eventually becomes atrophic, frequently appearing yellow, thus the epithet of "waxy disc."

Retinitis pigmentosa is classically bilateral, although the disease may be more advanced in one eye than in the other. Histologic studies indicate that retinitis pigmentosa is a disorder of the photoreceptors, primarily the rods. The pigmentary changes and vascular attenuation are probably secondary to the basic atrophic changes in the photoreceptors. The most universal and probably earliest symptom of retinitis pigmentosa is night blindness. The field defect that accompanies retinitis pigmentosa is classically a ring scotoma which corresponds to the equatorial pigmentation. Eventually, the ring scotoma progresses, and ultimately the entire visual field is lost, the central field being the last to go.

Figure 145. The typical appearance of *retinitis pigmentosa* is one of *bone spicule pigmentation* in the midperiphery of the fundus, a waxy appearance of the optic nerve head, marked narrowing, and attenuation of the vessels.

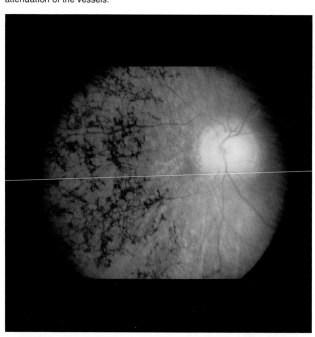

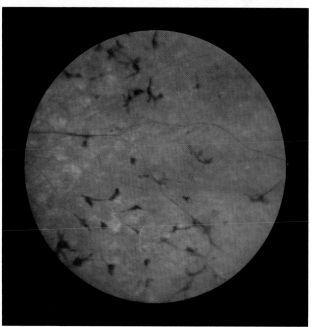

Figure 146. Retinitis pigmentosa. The retinal vessels are barely visible. The bone spicule pigmentation is sparse as compared to that in Figure 145.

The electroretinogram is consistently abnormal, even when the ophthalmoscopic signs are minimal. Retinitis pigmentosa has been associated with other systemic afflictions such as deaf-mutism, mental deficiency, and endocrine abnormalities. There is no known therapy, although light deprivation has been reported to slow the progress of the disease.

CHOROIDEREMIA

Choroideremia is a progressive, degenerative atrophy of the choroid. It is inherited as a sex-linked disease and is somewhat like retinitis pigmentosa in that both share symptoms of night blindness and long retention of central vision. However, retinitis pigmentosa is primarily a degenerative process of the retina, whereas choroideremia is primarily a degenerative disease of the choroid. These lesions usually occur in young males. A fine pigment mottling of the fundus is initially present; as the disease progresses, the ophthalmoscopic picture becomes classic (Figures 147 and 148). Large visible areas of sclera are traversed by a few choroidal vessels, and pigment clumping occurs. In the female carrier state, the appearance of the fundus is similar to that seen in very young affected male patients.

Figure 147. Choroideremia constitutes extensive atrophy of the choroid with loss of the overlying retinal function. In contrast to central areolar choroidal sclerosis, the choroidal vessels are not simply sclerosed, but tend to disappear entirely.

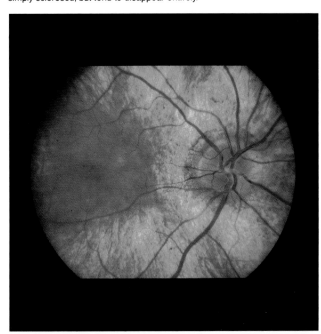

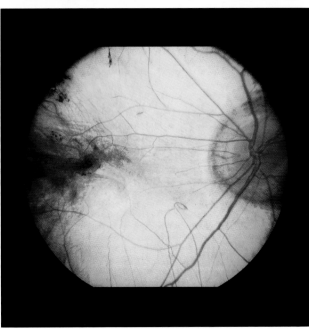

Figure 148. A more advanced case of choroideremia.

Figure 149A. *Gyrate atrophy* is a congenitally acquired progressive atrophic process affecting the choroid in well-circumscribed but eventually confluent areas. Retinal function diminishes progressively.

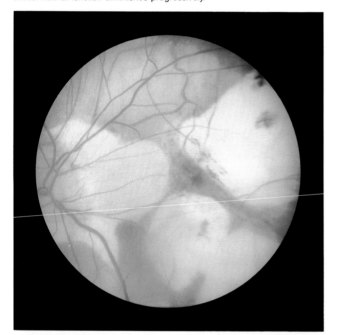

GYRATE ATROPHY

Gyrate atrophy is a degenerative process that involves both the choroid and the retina. Although considered to be related to choroideremia, it has a different pattern of inheritance, being recessive rather than sex-linked. Ophthalmoscopically, this condition is characterized by patchy atrophy of the choroid, starting in the equatorial region (Figure 149). This is accompanied by atrophy of the choriocapillaris and the larger choroidal blood vessels, resulting in large areas of visible sclera. The retinal blood vessels and optic nerve head usually remain normal. The presenting symptom is night blindness; the usual field abnormality is peripheral contraction. Central vision is spared until the late stages of the disorder.

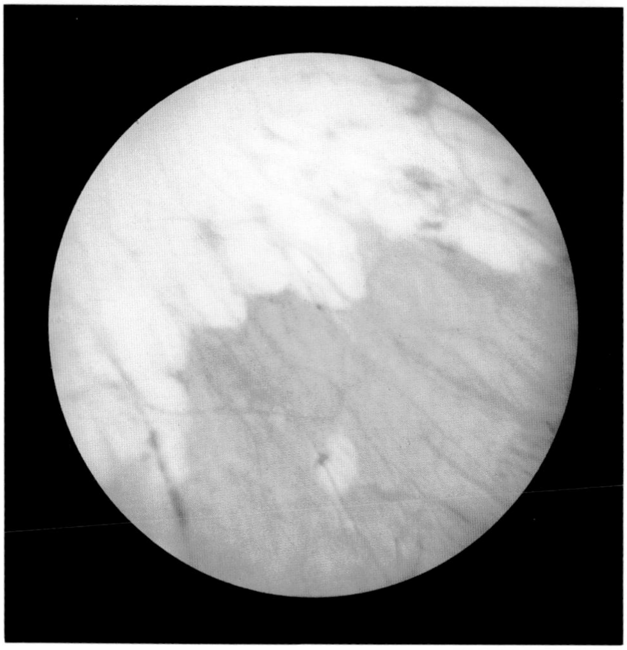

Figure 149B. Different view of the same fundus. A peripheral serrated margin of gyrate atrophy helps to distinguish it from the acquired visibility of sclera in high myopia (see Figure 49).

Folds, Striae, and Streaks

Figure 150A. *Choroidal folds* may occur as idiopathic phenomena.

CHOROIDAL FOLDS

Choroidal folds are easily detected ophthalmoscopi-cally, appearing as horizontal lines at the posterior pole. Although vertical folds are seen occasionally, they are much less common than the horizontal folds. The variable number of folds usually extend from above and below the disc toward the macula. Ophthalmo-scopically, one can observe the crests of the folds alter-nating with the troughs that usually run as parallel yellow and dark streaks (Figures 150 and 151). In some instances, the vision is affected by the distortion of the overlying photoreceptors. Fluorescein angiography delineates the folds, producing a characteristic picture of hyperfluorescence of the peaks while the troughs remain dark. Although choroidal folds are sometimes idiopathic, they are more often associated with orbital masses such as tumors, pseudotumors, Graves' oph-thalmopathy, intraocular choroidal tumors, and scleral buckling procedures for retinal detachments. Following an operation for uveitis or cataracts, if there is a decrease in the production of aqueous humor or a wound leak that produces hypotony, the choroid and retinal pig-ment epithelium may be thrown into folds. When the precipitating disease process is corrected, there may be regression of the choroidal folds and subsequent improvement in vision.

RETINAL STRIAE

Retinal striae affecting the posterior pole occur with retrolental fibroplasia, perforating injuries, and a few rare ocular inflammations of unknown cause. For ex-ample, extremely fine, generally horizontal, finger-print-like "reflexes" indicate a wrinkling of the internal limiting membrane on the retina's surface (Figure 152). Such abnormality may be a very subtle finding consti-tuting a challenge met only by careful examination of the macula through a well-dilated pupil. Little can be said regarding the cause of such wrinkling of the inter-

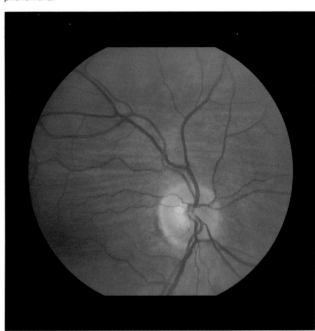

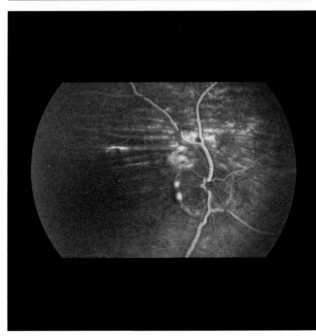

Figure 150B. Folds are best demonstrated by fluorescein angiography.

Figure 151. This 14-year-old girl had an encapsulated orbital hemangioma causing proptosis of the left eye, papilledema, and choroidal folds. The right fundus is normal, shown for comparison.

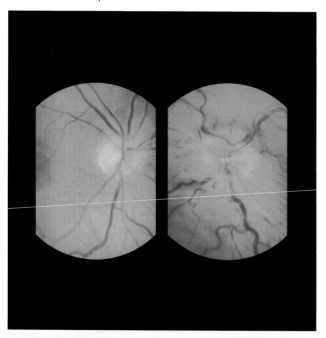

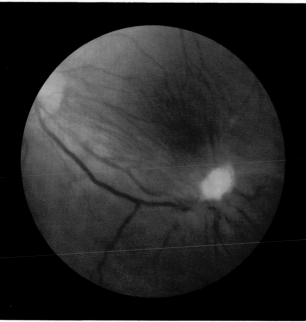

Figure 152. *Retinal striae* are delicate linear markings. These striae are not visible with fluorescein angiography, although they do cause distortion and tortuosity of the fine retinal vessels. Retinal tension lines result from superficial inflammatory lesions of the retina, often of unknown etiology.

nal limiting membrane. It is associated with increased tortuosity of the fine retinal vessels in the affected area. At times it is bilateral and occasionally the disease regresses spontaneously.

ANGIOID STREAKS

Angioid streaks are fundus findings originally thought to be caused by abnormal vasculature, hence, the misnomer, angioid. In fact, these streaks are cracks that occur along lines of stress in an abnormal Bruch's membrane rendered brittle by deposition of calcium or other heavy metals (Figures 153 and 154). Angioid streaks are maroon in lightly pigmented fundi and slate gray in non-Caucasians. Angioid streaks, when present in full array, have peripapillary interlacement and radial extensions reaching toward the equator. The streaks taper as they extend peripherally and their margins have jigsaw-puzzle contours. Since they are located posterior to the retina, the overlying pattern of retinal vessels is entirely normal.

At times, a typical *peau d'orange* appearance of the fundus is seen, representing diffuse abnormality of the retinal pigment epithelium (Figure 155). Hemorrhagic macular degeneration (Figure 156) is a common accompaniment and in some patients may precede ophthalmoscopically visible streaks. As the chorioretinal degenerative changes slowly progress, there is proliferation of fibrovascular membranes from the choroid into the posterior retina, causing certain eventual loss of central vision through hemorrhagic macular degeneration. No therapy has proved effective.

88

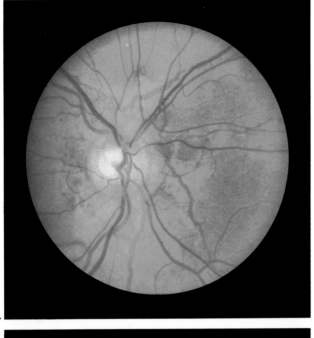

153.

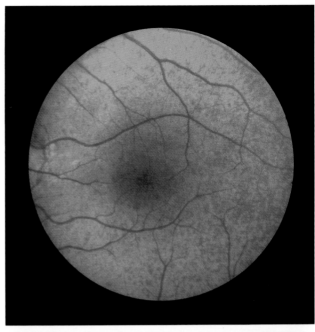

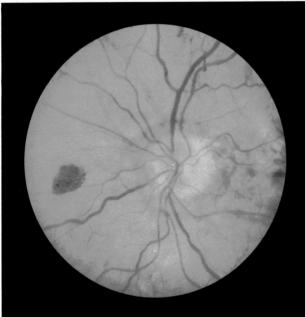

154A.

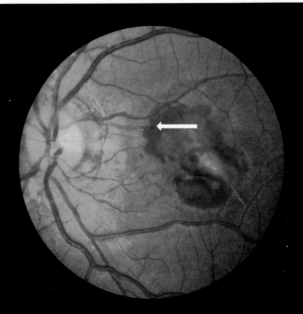

Figure 153. *Angioid streaks* are radially arranged linear markings that underlie the retinal vasculature and often join in a peripapillary encirclement. These streaks are present at the nasal margin of the nerve head in this illustration.

Figure 154A. An array of angioid streaks is visible and can be differentiated from the overlying retinal vasculature. The optic nerve head demonstrates a pseudopapilledema resulting from frequently present hyaline bodies of the disc.

Figure 154B. An artist's rendition of the pathology of angioid streaks. Note in the cut section of the retina that the streaks constitute cracks in Bruch's membrane (dark blue color) which separates the retina from the choroid. Extensive scarring from disciform degeneration of the macula is also illustrated.

Figure 155. A *peau d'orange* appearance of the fundus is commonly found in patients having angioid streaks.

Figure 156. In Negroes, angioid streaks appear slate gray (arrow) and are more easily recognized than the maroon-colored linear markings in Caucasians (see Figure 153). Hemorrhagic macular degeneration is a common accompaniment of angioid streaks in pseudoxanthoma elasticum, Paget's disease of bone, and sickle cell disease.

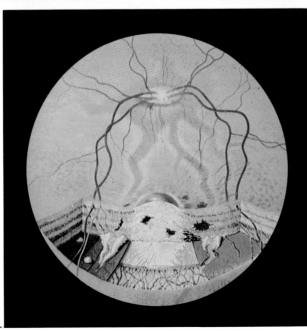

154B.

Phakomatoses

Phakoma is a term meaning "mother spot." The phakomatoses include a group of congenital diseases manifested by skin lesions and associated hamartomas of
other organs. A *hamartoma* is a tumor composed of
persistent embryologic tissue native to that particular
organ that only rarely undergoes neoplastic transforma-
tion. Some of these conditions have minimal cutaneous
involvement and are characterized by the conspicuous
hamartomas. The phakomatoses to be discussed and
illustrated are tuberous sclerosis, neurofibromatosis,
and angiomatosis retinae.

TUBEROUS SCLEROSIS

Tuberous sclerosis is a genetic disorder of unknown
etiology, characterized by hamartomas arising in the
skin, nervous system, heart, kidney, and eye. Clinical
manifestations of this syndrome include adenoma
sebaceum of the skin, epilepsy, and mental retardation.
Children born with the disease usually appear normal
at birth and only gradually develop clinical stigmata.
Seizures and psychomotor retardation are early manifestations. Classically, facial adenoma sebaceum becomes prominent in later childhood. The facial lesions,
although called adenoma sebaceum, are actually angio-
fibromas with secondary involvement of the sebaceous
glands. Other common diagnostic lesions include sub-
epidermal fibrosis, and subungual and periungual
fibromas. Radiographically, one may see calcified cerebral astrocytes referred to as "brain stones." Although
adenoma sebaceum, mental retardation, and epilepsy
are hallmarks of this disease, they each may progress at
different rates and may not parallel each other. When
all three of these clinical expressions are present, the
diagnosis is readily apparent. In young patients, or
when only one clinical manifestation is obvious, the
presence of cutaneous or retinal lesions confirms the
diagnosis.

The ocular lesion of tuberous sclerosis is a hamarto-

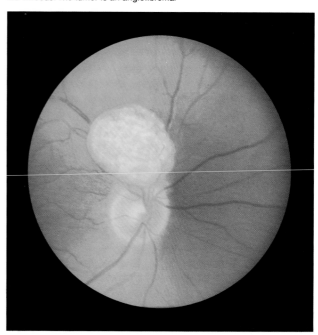

Figure 157. The ocular manifestations of *tuberous sclerosis* include the classical appearance of this hamartomatous tumor extending from the retina into the vitreous. The tumor is an angiofibroma.

ma of the retinal nerve fiber layer appearing as a smooth
elevation of the retina. Multiple lesions may be found
at the posterior pole. At puberty, these lesions may un-
dergo calcific degeneration forming an ophthalmoscopic *mulberry lesion* (Figure 157). This gross hamartomatous proliferation may impair vision. There is very
little that can be done for these patients. Diagnostically,
these lesions have to be differentiated from retinoblastomas.

NEUROFIBROMATOSIS

Neurofibromatosis is a hereditary, apparently autosomal dominant disorder involving the skin, nervous
system, bones, endocrine glands, and eyes. The typical
clinical picture consists of multiple areas of increased
skin pigmentation, accompanied by dermal and neural
tumors of various sizes, involving the central nervous
system as well as the cranial and spinal nerves.

The most frequent ocular manifestations of neurofibromatosis are lid lesions. The eyelid plexiform fibroma feels like a bag of worms on palpation and may produce a disfiguring unilateral ptosis. Solitary tumors as well as café-au-lait spots and cutaneous nevi are also found on the lids. Orbital neurofibromata may be associated with a large defect in the orbital bones and pulsating exophthalmos. Slit-lamp examination of an affected eye often reveals neurofibromata of the iris appearing as small brown nodules. The classic ocular manifestation is an optic nerve glioma which occurs in approximately 15% of patients with neurofibromatosis. These gliomas may produce proptosis and eventually optic atrophy (Figure 158). The orbital and lid fibromata are not very amenable to surgical extirpation. Gliomas of the optic nerve are difficult to remove surgically without sacrificing the entire eye, and even then the tumor may extend back to the chiasm.

ANGIOMATOSIS RETINAE

Von Hippel's syndrome, or angiomatosis retinae, is one of the classic phakomas characterized by hamartomatous lesions of the retina and central nervous system, and is frequently associated with cysts of the kidneys, liver, and pancreas. The inheritance pattern of von Hippel's disease is thought to be autosomal dominant with incomplete penetrance. The central nervous system lesion, which occurs in 25% of patients, is a cystic hemangioblastoma of the cerebellum. When angiomatosis retinae is associated with a cerebellar hemangioblastoma, the condition is referred to as von Hippel-Lindau disease. Recently, a significant incidence of pheochromocytomas has been reported in patients with angiomatosis (this is also true with neurofibromatosis).

The retinal tumors are considered to be hamartomatous lesions of the entire vascular bed, involving the arteriole, capillary, and efferent veins. These tumors usually begin at the capillary level with secondary changes occurring in the afferent and efferent vessels.

Figure 158. Neurofibromatosis can affect the eye in many forms. This patient had an extensive tumor in the orbit and marked proptosis of the eye leading to ischemia of the optic nerve with subsequent atrophy, marked narrowing and sheathing of the arterioles, and pigment proliferation similar to retinitis pigmentosa. The latter is the result of interruption of the blood supply from the posterior ciliary arteries which supply the choroidal circulation. (Green discoloration is an artifact that commonly occurs when a fundus photograph is taken through a small pupil.)

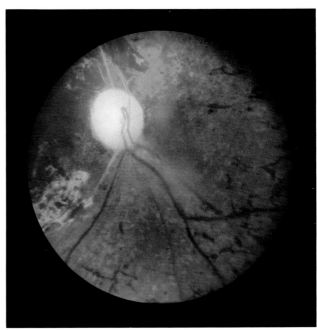

The ophthalmoscopic finding consists of large globular, flesh-colored tumors associated with dilated afferent and efferent vessels (Figure 159). In this condition there is frequently associated subretinal exudation and a secondary glial proliferation. Although the tumors may occur anywhere, they are seen classically near the posterior pole and at times in the peripapillary area. The tumors are bilateral in 50% of the cases. Incipient, or early, tumors may appear as small vascular abnormalities in the peripheral retina. These retinal tumors may be treated effectively by photocoagulation or cryotherapy.

The differential diagnosis includes the Wyburn-Mason syndrome (Figure 160) with its extraordinary array of vascular abnormality and related central nervous system involvement.

Figure 159A. A patient with angiomatosis retinae has hard exudates at the macula, nasal to the optic nerve head. A retinal angioma is located superotemporal to the disc.

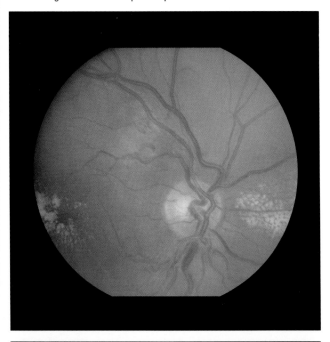

Figure 159C. Far inferiorly (and in the same fundus), a large angioma and dilated vasculature are shown.

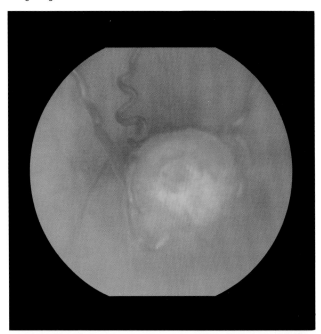

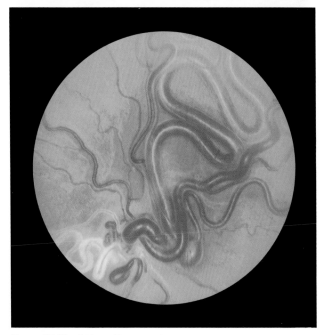

Figure 159B. The same fundus shows the disc and the inferonasal region where vascular tortuosity and more exudates occur.

Figure 160. The *Wyburn-Mason syndrome* is illustrated by the tortuous fundus vessels with arteriovenous communication and complete loss of the normal vascular pattern and normal A/V ratio. Arteriovenous malformations of the retina, orbit, and midbrain occur in this syndrome.

ACKNOWLEDGEMENTS

Figure 1. Adapted from art by Sharon Weilbacher

Figure 6. Painting by Howard Bartner. Previously published in Bartner H and Paton D: A Model Eye for Instruction in Indirect Ophthalmoscopy. *Annals of Ophthalmology;* Aug-Sept, 1969; Figure 2, page 45. Reprinted with permission of publisher.

Figures 15, 23, 65, 37, 103, 116B. Dan M. Gordon, Scope® Monograph on Fundamentals of Ophthalmoscopy. The Upjohn Company, Kalamazoo, Michigan, 1973.

Figures 102A, 102B. Alice McPherson MD, Houston, Texas, supplied these photographs of a diabetic retina before and after treatment with the argon laser.

Figures 119, 133, 134. Published in Paton D and Goldberg MF: *Management of Ocular Injuries.* Philadelphia, WB Saunders Co., 1976. Reprinted with permission of the publisher.

Figure 154B. Painting by Joel Schechter, published in Paton D: *The Relation of Angioid Streaks to Systemic Disease.* Springfield, Charles C. Thomas, Publisher, 1972. Reprinted with permission of publisher.